ETHICS IN EPIDEMIOLOGY AND PUBLIC HEALTH PRACTICE

Collected Works

Second Edition

Steven S. Coughlin, Ph.D.

D0469050

American Public Health Association
800 I Street, NW
Washington, DC 20001-3710
www.apha.org

Georges C. Benjamin, MD, FACP, *Executive Director*
Carlos Castillo–Salgado, MD, JD, MPH, DrPH, *Publications Board Liaison*

Printed and bound in the United States of America

Interior Design and Typesetting: Manila Typesetting Company
Cover Design: Jennifer Strauss
Printing and Binding: Sheridan Books, Inc.

Library of Congress Cataloging-in-Publication Data

Coughlin, Steven S. (Steven Scott), 1957-
  Ethics in epidemiology and public health practice : collected works / Steven S. Coughlin. – 2nd ed.
  p. ; cm.
  Includes bibliographical references and index.
  ISBN-13: 978-0-87553-193-9
  ISBN-10: 0-87553-193-8
  1. Epidemiologist–Professional ethics. 2. Public health personnel–Professional ethics. I. American Public Health Association. II. Title.
  [DNLM: 1. Epidemiology. 2. Ethics, Professional. 3. Public Health. WA 21 C854e 2009]
  RA652.C68 2009
  174'.2–dc22

                          2009039468

ISBN 13:978-0-87553-193-9
ISBN 10: 0-87553-193-8
1500/10/2009

TABLE OF CONTENTS

PREFACE

This anthology of articles on ethics in epidemiology and public health practice substantially updates and expands the topics dealt with in the first edition of this book. The topics covered in this second edition include ethical issues in epidemiologic research, public health practice, ethics instruction, and ethics guidelines for epidemiologists. Several theoretical and applied aspects of public health ethics at public health agencies and institutions are also dealt with, including general ethical principles and organizational ethics.

Since the publication of the first edition of this book, there have been several notable developments in ethics, epidemiology, and public health practice. These include the publication of scholarly articles outlining the principles and terrain of public health ethics, new books on public health ethics and closely related topics, and the release of important papers on ethical issues in public health ethics (e.g., a consultation paper prepared by the Nuffield Council on Bioethics in Great Britain). However, few resources have been available that articulate ethical issues in both epidemiologic research and in public health practice.

This book would not have been possible without the support and encouragement of many friends and colleagues who share my enthusiasm for ethics. I would particularly like to thank Drue Barrett, Richard Dixon, and other members of the Centers for Disease Control and Prevention Public Health Ethics Committee; Germaine Buck, Dixie Snider Jr., Colin Soskolne, Douglas Weed, and other past and present members of the American College of Epidemiology Ethics and Standards of Practice Committee; and Tom Beauchamp, Gayle Clutter, Mary Hutton, and faculty and students at the Rollins School of Public Health at Emory University. In addition, I am most grateful to Norman Giesbrecht and Carlos Castillo-Salgado, who represented the American Public Health Association (APHA) Publications Board, Carrie Mercadante, APHA Book Production Coordinator, and Nina Tristani, APHA Director of Publications.

PART I

INTRODUCTION

Epidemiology, the study of the distribution and determinants of disease in human populations, is a foundational science in public health. The results of epidemiologic studies contribute to generalizable knowledge by clarifying the causes of diseases, by combining epidemiologic data with information from other disciplines (e.g., genetics, industrial hygiene, health education), by evaluating the consistency of epidemiologic data with etiological hypotheses about causation, and by providing the basis for evaluating procedures for health promotion and prevention and public health practices. Public health practice includes such essential public health services and functions as outbreak investigations, program evaluations, public health surveillance, many disease prevention and control activities, and emergency preparedness and response.

The articles included in this section highlight a number of important ethics concepts and issues in epidemiology and public health practice including core values in the field. The examination of core values can help illuminate ethical precepts while highlighting positive aspects of ethics. Of key interest are mission statements for public health institutions, preambles to ethics guidelines for epidemiologists, and results obtained from ethics surveys of epidemiologists and representatives of public health institutions. Viewed in this light, professional ethics has little to do with watching out for wrongdoing or reprimanding practitioners, and more to do with the clarification of a variety of ethical norms and duties of epidemiologists and other public health professionals, including issues about which reasonable people may disagree. Prospectively defining the mission and core values of an organization may help to resolve conflicts among competing values, particularly if staff at various levels are involved in the process. Many public health organizations have taken measures to develop statements of their mission, vision, and core values, and to communicate those statements to their employees. The aspirational and inspirational aspects of an organization's vision statement may help public health professionals and other employees understand more clearly what the organization would like to become. Mission statements articulate how the vision will be accomplished. In the readings that follow, examples of such statements are provided from leading public health agencies, and biomedical research institutions and universities.

The second article included in this section highlights a number of unresolved ethical questions in epidemiology. Other unresolved questions highlighted in the recent literature on research ethics include how best to balance privacy protections such as the Health Insurance Portability and Accountability Act of 1996 (HIPAA) requirements with the need for efficient research studies on important health topics [1]. Leading epidemiologists have noted that HIPAA requirements may serve as a barrier to some forms of epidemiologic research, and they do not protect identifiable research data that are not considered protected health information. Unless the investigators have obtained a certificate of confidentiality, research data may also be subject to subpoena by a court of law. Institutional review boards (IRBs), which have an important role in protecting the privacy of research subjects and maintaining the confidentiality of data, may require investigators to obtain a certificate of confidentiality for studies involving the collection of sensitive data such as information about drug use, or history of HIV/AIDS or a genetic disorder. Another example of an unresolved issue in human subjects research is the ongoing debate about the extent to which research participants are adequately protected by existing safeguards or whether the regulatory system for protecting human subjects is overregulated. Some critics have charged that IRBs devote an increasing amount of time to activities of marginal utility (e.g., meticulously documenting compliance with federal rules and regulations) and that this focus on minutiae may distract them from more important substantive issues. Other examples of unresolved ethical questions in epidemiology arise in deliberations about whether associations with suspected etiologic factors are causal, and how much evidence is sufficient to warrant public health agencies to intervene to protect public health [2].

1.   The Health Insurance Portability and Accountability Act of 1996. Available at http://www.
      hhs.gov/ocr/privacy/index.html.
2.   Weed, D.L. Toward a Philosophy of Epidemiology. In: Coughlin, S.S., T.L. Beauchamp, and
      D.L. Weed, editors, *Ethics and Epidemiology* (2nd ed.). New York, NY: Oxford University
      Press (2009).

CHAPTER 1

ETHICS IN EPIDEMIOLOGY AT THE END OF THE TWENTIETH CENTURY. ETHICS, VALUES, AND MISSION STATEMENTS

Steven S. Coughlin

Important advances occurred in ethics and epidemiology in the closing decades of the twentieth century [1, 2]. These advances include explications of the societal importance of epidemiologic research and practice, clarifications of the ethical duties of epidemiologists, and the increasing integration of ethics into the professional life of epidemiologists [3–12]. These developments in ethics are not isolated events. Rather, they have occurred in conjunction with historical events: improvements in institutional and regulatory safeguards for protecting human subjects, rising public concern over the privacy and confidentiality of medical records, the onset of the AIDS epidemic, and the emergence of molecular epidemiology, to name a few.

One sign of the increased attention to ethics and values in epidemiology in recent years is the development of ethics guidelines for epidemiologists and policy statements on data sharing, privacy and confidentiality protection, deoxyribonucleic acid (DNA) testing for disease susceptibility, and other issues [6–10, 13–15]. Courses on ethics in epidemiology and public health have also been initiated at several institutions that train public health professionals [16–19]. In addition, the number of publications on ethical issues in epidemiology has increased [20–23]. Indeed, all these developments have likely contributed to the increasing recognition of epidemiology as a distinct profession [2, 12].

The focus of these developments (ethics guidelines, curricula, and publications) has often been on identifying and communicating ethical rules and duties and on controversial or still-evolving ethical precepts (e.g., the extent to which epidemiologists should engage in public health advocacy) [24–26]. Ethical problems, such as conflicts of interest and scientific misconduct, have also been dealt with [27–33]. Less attention has been given to core values in epidemiology, even though an examination of core values may help to clarify ethical precepts in epidemiology while highlighting positive aspects of professional ethics.

To identify and clarify basic scientific values in the field, I examine core values in epidemiology and public health as reflected in mission statements for public health institutions, preambles to ethics guidelines for epidemiologists, and results obtained from ethics surveys. Professional values are discussed in relation to an important controversy in

"Ethics in Epidemiology at the End of the Twentieth Century. Ethics, Values, and Mission Statements" originally appeared in *Epidemiologic Reviews (2000):22:169–175. Used with permission of Oxford University Press, Inc.*

contemporary epidemiology: whether epidemiology has failed to sustain its commitment to public health. Finally, I discuss future directions of ethics and values in epidemiology.

Core Values in Epidemiology

Core values are fundamental ethical and scientific precepts (i.e., basic scientific values) that are consistent with and provide support for the mission and purpose of the profession. In the case of epidemiology, the mission is to acquire new scientific information that can be used to maintain, enhance, and promote the public's health [9, 34–36]. Widely held and accepted core values exist within the profession of epidemiology. Nevertheless, individual epidemiologists may hold different opinions about core values, and the values in the profession may gradually change or evolve over time [36]. Core values in epidemiology are closely related to core values in the broader field of public health. As Barry Levy explained in his American Public Health Association presidential address in November 1997, "Values define us as a group of public health professionals; values drew many of us into public health in the first place" ([37], p. 191).

Published accounts suggest that, like other scientists, epidemiologists accept ideals of free inquiry and the pursuit of knowledge and that they uphold the values of improving the public's health by applying scientific knowledge [5, 22]. The manner in which these core values guide epidemiologic research and practice is shaped by societal values and by the personal values of individual epidemiologists. As Susser et al. [5] noted, an examination of ethics in epidemiology is an examination of the way in which the values of science and its potential benefits to public health are balanced against the values of individuals and communities. Other values within the profession that may be less fundamental but nevertheless important (e.g., the value of establishing partnerships between academic and public health practice institutions), and epidemiologic duties and virtues (e.g., the obligation that epidemiologists have to respect the autonomy of persons) further shape the influence of core values.

Core values can be distinguished from duties and ethical rules, which are more specific and tied to specific contexts (e.g., the rule that research protocols involving human subjects should be submitted for ethical review by an IRB) [11, 38]. Duties are those obligations epidemiologists hold to various parties, such as subjects, society, funding sources, employers, and colleagues [7, 11]. Core values can also be distinguished from epidemiologic virtues that are often aspirational and grounded in professional character (e.g., truth telling, objectivity, scientific excellence [11, 39]). Whereas epidemiologic values are not based in any particular moral theory, virtues are an important aspect of virtue ethics, a moral theory that emphasizes the character and moral motivation of the agent (person) rather than the actions taken by the person [39, 40].

Our understanding of core values and specific ethical rules and duties in epidemiology is shaped by contemporary discussions about ethical issues arising in biomedical research, such as issues arising in genetics research, how best to protect participants in placebo-controlled trials, and guidelines for conducting studies in developing countries [15, 41–43].

Epidemiologic Values Reflected in Mission Statements

Core values and other values in the profession are reflected in mission statements that have been drafted by an increasing number of epidemiology professional societies. For example, the mission statement of the American College of Epidemiology states that it is a professional organization that serves the interests of its members (i.e., epidemiologists) through sponsorship of scientific meetings, publications, and educational activities; it recognizes outstanding contributions to the field and advocates for issues pertinent to epidemiology [44]. Thus, the college highlights the value of disseminating and sharing scientific information, providing continuing professional education, promoting scientific excellence, and advancing the profession. The mission statement of the International Society for Environmental Epidemiology states that the society provides a forum for discussing problems unique to the study of health and the environment. With membership open to environmental epidemiologists and other scientists worldwide, the society provides a variety of forums for discussions, critical reviews, collaborations, and education on issues of environmental exposures and their human health effects [45]. These activities include annual meetings; newsletters; workshops; and liaisons with academic, governmental, intergovernmental, nonprofit, and business institutions. Thus, in addition to the dissemination of scientific information and continuing professional education, the society upholds the value of international and interdisciplinary scientific collaboration and links with stakeholders outside the profession.

Epidemiology values are also reflected in statements drafted for public health institutions. For example, the U.S. Centers for Disease Control and Prevention (CDC) statement of core values emphasizes the need for CDC employees to act decisively and compassionately in service to people's health and to ensure that CDC research and services are based on sound science and meet genuine public needs [46]. Respect for persons, cultural diversity, honesty, scientific integrity, and professional excellence are also emphasized in the statement. The CDC has employees from many disciplines, including epidemiology, the basic sciences, and other public health professions. The National Institutes of Health, a federal biomedical research institution in the United States, also have a multidisciplinary workforce. Their mission statement emphasizes science in pursuit of fundamental knowledge about the nature and behavior of living systems and the application of that knowledge to extend healthy life and reduce the burdens of illness and disability [47]. The goals include creative discoveries and innovative research strategies; their application to protect and improve health; and scientific integrity, public accountability, and social responsibility in the conduct of science.

Many schools of public health (which include epidemiology training programs) have developed mission statements. The goals of the University of Texas at Houston School of Public Health, for example, emphasize education, research, community service, and the importance of public health values [48]:

> The mission of the school is to improve and sustain the health of people by providing the highest quality graduate education, research, and community service for Texas, the nation, and internationally. The school provides the citizens of Texas the opportunity for quality graduate education in the basic disciplines and practices of public health, extends knowledge of these disciplines, and assists public health practitioners. The mission emphasizes:
>
> *Education*—The school's first responsibility is to provide present and future practitioners, teachers, and scientists the highest quality graduate education in the theory and practice of public health. Its educational philosophy is based on the premise that education is a lifelong process and that, while the school

offers resources and guidance, the fundamental responsibility for each person's education resides with the individual, with guidance and support of the faculty. The school teaches public health values and a diversity of skills in the physical, biologic, behavioral, and analytic sciences needed by public health practitioners today. The school is committed to maintaining a broad perspective of health, disease, and the health care system.

Research—The school is committed to the pursuit of knowledge which enhances both the theory and practice of public health. Faculty support and engage in research directed toward such activities as health promotion, environmental health, disease control, and health care delivery.

Community Service—The faculty seek to provide service to local, state, national, and international health agencies that is consistent with the school's instructional and research commitments. The school develops public policy, contributes to the activities of these agencies, and enhances the well-being of the public.

Public health practice, public health research, and service to local, state, national, and international agencies and communities are also highlighted in the mission statement.

Epidemiologic Values Reflected in Ethics Guidelines

A number of sets of ethics guidelines for epidemiologists have been proposed [6–9]. Guidelines drafted by the International Epidemiological Association include a preamble defining the purpose of epidemiology; a statement of core values in epidemiology; a summary of basic principles of biomedical ethics; and various sections outlining the obligations of epidemiologists to individuals, communities, colleagues, employers and funding agencies, and the profession [6]. The guidelines state, "We who practice epidemiology are concerned with the health of all population groups. Our role is to identify interventions likely to restore, maintain and improve health . . . . As public health professionals, we have an obligation to communities . . ." [6]. Other values are implicit in the discussion of professional obligations of epidemiologists. For example, the association's draft guidelines indicate that epidemiology is primarily concerned with providing service to communities and that epidemiologists are frequently drawn to the problems of disempowered communities. Cultural variations in values are also discussed in the guidelines.

Ethics guidelines proposed by the Industrial Epidemiology Forum provide an account of the obligations of epidemiologists to research subjects, society, employers and funding agencies, and colleagues [7]. Although the guidelines are written in the form of professional obligations or duties, they do provide some information about core values in the field. For example, the accompanying commentary states, "The principles in these guidelines presume that there is no absolute right to scientific investigation even if scientific knowledge stands to be advanced appreciably. The advancement of knowledge is a worthy pursuit, but it is not so valuable as to provide a sufficient justification in all cases for overriding competing values such as privacy, confidentiality, and protection against risk" ([7], p. 157S). Thus, the guidelines highlight the value that epidemiologists and society place on general ethical principles (e.g., avoiding harm, providing benefits, balancing benefits against risks, respecting personal autonomy, and protecting privacy and confidentiality).

The Council for International Organizations for Medical Sciences' "International Guidelines for Ethical Review of Epidemiological Studies" [8] addresses similar issues.

These guidelines draw a distinction between epidemiologic research and routine practice and consider the problems associated with obtaining informed consent and respecting cultural differences in ethics and values in some epidemiologic studies. The guidelines note, "Ethical issues often arise as a result of conflict among competing sets of values, such as in the field of public health, the conflict between the rights of individuals, and the needs of communities" ([8], p. 250).

Ethics guidelines for environmental epidemiologists drafted by Soskolne and Light [9] summarize the mission and core values of environmental epidemiology. They note that the mission of environmental epidemiology is to maintain, enhance, and promote health in communities worldwide by identifying or evaluating environmental hazards. Soskolne and Light [9] also note that environmental epidemiologists contribute to scientific knowledge about environmental risks and environmentally induced diseases and that they protect public health at the local, regional, national, and global levels.

The Italian Epidemiological Association and the American College of Epidemiology refined and updated ethics guidelines for epidemiologists. These documents are likely to further contribute to our understanding of ethics and values in epidemiology [17, 49].

Ethics guidelines for epidemiologists can be considered within the broader context of regional and international guidelines for biomedical researchers, which have also been periodically revised and updated [50, 51].

Epidemiologic Values Reflected in Results from Ethics Surveys

Ethics surveys have provided information about the ethical interests and concerns of epidemiologists and about core values in the field. Surveys to date have targeted epidemiologists and other public health professionals, public health students, and institutions that train public health professionals [19, 52–55].

Soskolne et al. [52] conducted an international ethics survey in 1994 among environmental epidemiologists. The participants were reached through mailings from the International Society for Environmental Epidemiology, the Italian Epidemiological Association, and the Global Environmental Epidemiology Network (managed by the Office of Global and Integrated Environmental Health of the World Health Organization, Geneva, Switzerland). The response rate was about 30% for the International Society for Environmental Epidemiology and 19% for the Global Environmental Epidemiology Network. A total of 346 returned questionnaires were available for analysis. The survey focused on statements of ethical values and principles that were grouped into nine major areas. The greatest disagreement concerned the role of the environmental epidemiologist as a "dispassionate scientist" or a "passionate advocate"; other disagreement revolved around whether environmental epidemiology is an applied science or a basic science and whether environmental epidemiologists should be committed to influencing society in ways that maximize the likelihood of "health for all." Thus, the results suggest that different opinions among environmental epidemiologists exist about certain ethical precepts and professional obligations. The differences may reflect a lack of consensus about the mission of environmental epidemiology and core values in the field or, alternatively, a measurement problem (e.g., ambiguity in the wording of the questionnaire).

To obtain input from practicing epidemiologists on ethics guidelines, the American College of Epidemiology's Ethics and Standards of Practice Committee developed a questionnaire [53]. The survey was conducted among a random sample of 300 North American members of the American College of Epidemiology, the Society for Epidemiologic Research, and the American Heart Association Council on Epidemiology and Prevention. The response rate was 88% (265 respondents). The majority of respondents agreed that any new ethics guidelines should address the goals and purposes of epidemiologic research that (according to questionnaire items for which there was good agreement) include "providing a rational basis for improving public health," "increasing scientific knowledge," and "establishing, guiding, changing public policy." There was less agreement among the respondents about the need for guidelines to address the "use of study results to advocate change in values or customs."

Professional Values and Epidemiology's Commitment to Public Health

The 1988 report *The Future of Public Health* by the Institute of Medicine observed, "public health professionals rely on expert knowledge derived from such areas as epidemiology and biostatistics to identify and deal with the health needs of whole populations. A central tenet of their professional ethic is commitment to use this knowledge to fulfill the public interest in reducing human suffering and enhancing the quality of life" ([56], p. 4). The report also noted that knowledge and values remain decisive elements in the shaping of public health practice. Similar sentiments were expressed by Krieger and Zierler [57] who, as epidemiologists, share a vision of reducing human suffering by generating beneficial knowledge.

In the past decade, there has been extensive debate about whether epidemiology has lost its commitment to public health [58–62]. Terris [59] argued that, as a result of a shift of epidemiologic research from health departments to schools of public health, epidemiology has withdrawn from the community (e.g., fewer field studies and more secondary analyses of existing data) and that concern with the methodology of data manipulation—rather than with the solution of disease problems—has grown. He noted "an orientation geared more to the goal of 'publish or perish' than to the goal of preventing disease and death" ([59], p. 913).

Some leading epidemiologists have criticized epidemiology subspecialties, such as clinical epidemiology and molecular epidemiology, because of a perceived lack of a population perspective and public health orientation. For example, Last [63] argued against the uncritical enthusiasm with which clinical epidemiology has been embraced by many medical schools. He was concerned about a particular definition of epidemiology: the use of clinical experience to inform and guide decisions about the care of individual patients. Last argued, "such a narrow view of epidemiology would sadden the founders of the Epidemiological Society of London, most of whom were public health workers and saw epidemiology as a discipline that existed primarily to protect and promote the public health" ([63], p. 160). Of course, many clinical epidemiologists and epidemiologists in other subspecialties may uphold public health values [36].

Susser and Susser [61, 62] called for a return to public health values and for a paradigm shift from the current emphasis on individual risk factors for disease to a new ecologic approach ("eco-epidemiology") that encompasses many levels of organization, including molecular, individual, and societal. Gori [64] observed that the two approaches (eco-epidemiology and the present paradigm, which emphasizes individual risk factors for disease) are complimentary rather than opposed. In a commentary about "black box epidemiology," Weed [65] argued that epidemiologists need a common set of values and that they lack consensus about their obligation to public health. He concluded that epidemiologists should embrace a systems theory approach.

Although epidemiologists remain divided about the need for a new scientific paradigm in their field, the debate has drawn attention to the need for a sustained epidemiologic commitment to public health. To some commentators, present efforts in epidemiology to address public health problems are insufficient. Echoing concerns by other authors [57–62], Pearce and McKinlay [66] argued that epidemiologists should pay more attention to the real determinants of health at the upstream population level (including socioeconomic, cultural, and political factors), address the most important public health questions, and use appropriate methods to address these questions. Such scientific arguments are founded in social concerns and in core values in epidemiology and public health.

Ethics, Values, and Future Directions in Epidemiology

One future direction in epidemiology is likely to be the further development of curricula on public health ethics for epidemiology graduate students, including coursework on the ethics of epidemiologic research and practice [16–19, 55, 67]. The Council on Education for Public Health criteria for graduate schools of public health in the United States emphasize public health values, concepts, and ethics, but the criteria do not currently require ethics instruction. Courses on public health ethics provide students with the conceptual abilities and decision-making skills they need to deal successfully with ethical issues in their own research and practice [18]. The cognitive aspects of ethics that can be taught include the identification of the ethical commitments of epidemiologic research and practice, the application of concepts and methods for ethical decision-making to actual cases, and critical reflection about personal values and obligations as a public health professional [18, 39]. Small group discussion of ethics cases, including important historical cases such as the Tuskegee Syphilis Study, is an important part of such coursework [54]. Core values in epidemiology and public health are often informally transmitted through informal teaching and mentoring of students and fellows. Schools of public health and academic departments of epidemiology can be seen as communities with their own culture and subculture; students and fellows are taught what is valued in that culture and are provided opportunities to internalize the core values [68].

Future directions in epidemiology are also likely to include the development of mission statements, statements of core values, and ethics guidelines for epidemiology specialties, such as molecular epidemiology, reproductive and perinatal epidemiology, and public health practice [2]. Such efforts contribute to the further recognition of epidemiology subspecialties as distinct subdisciplines while reinforcing their commitment to public health. Mission statements and statements of core values may also contribute to efforts to educate the public and stakeholders about the societal importance of epidemiology.

Another possible direction is the further incorporation of epidemiologic perspectives into policy statements and regulations that deal with the protection of human subjects, the privacy and confidentiality of medical records, and genetic testing [14, 15]. For example, distinctions have not always been drawn between highly penetrant disease susceptibility genes and more common genetic polymorphisms in developing ethical rules for genetic testing carried out as part of research protocols [69].

Substantial attention has been given to issues surrounding the privacy and confidentiality of medical records, data sharing, and linkage of large databases for the purposes of health research [13, 14, 70]. In view of recent legal and regulatory developments in these areas and technological refinements, such as the increased use of health information systems and the Internet [71, 72], epidemiologists are likely to continue to face professional challenges related to these important topics for the foreseeable future.

Finally, more attention will likely be given to ethics and values in public health practice and to ways to resolve conflicts between professional values and community values [73–75]. The ethics of public health practice have often been neglected in the literature on ethics and epidemiology compared with issues that arise in epidemiologic research, but recent articles and presentations at scientific meetings suggest that increasing attention is being devoted to these important issues.

Acknowledgment

The findings and conclusions in this article are those of the author and do not necessarily reflect the official position of the CDC.

References

1. Coughlin, S.S., and T.L. Beauchamp. Historical Foundations. In: Coughlin S.S., and T.L. Beauchamp, editors, *Ethics and Epidemiology*. New York, NY: Oxford University Press 5–23.
2. Coughlin, S.S. Advancing Professional Ethics in Epidemiology. *J Epidemiol Biostat* (1996): 1:71–77.
3. Gordis, L., E. Gold, and R. Seltser. Privacy Protection in Epidemiologic and Medical Research: A Challenge and Responsibility. *Am J Epidemiol* (1977):105:163–168.
4. Cann, C.I., and K.J. Rothman. IRBs and Epidemiologic Research: How Inappropriate Restrictions Hamper Studies. *IRB* (1984):6:5–7.
5. Susser, M., Z. Stein, and J. Kline. Ethics in Epidemiology. *Ann Am Acad Polit Soc Sci* (1978):437:128–141.
6. International Epidemiological Association. Ethical Guidelines for Epidemiologists (draft). In: *Epidemiology Section Newsletter*. Washington, D.C.: American Public Health Association, winter (1990).
7. Beauchamp, T.L., R.R. Cook, W.E. Fayerweather, et al. Ethical Guidelines for Epidemiologists. *J Clin Epidemiol* (1991):44:151S–169S.
8. Council for International Organizations of Medical Sciences. International Guidelines for Ethical Review of Epidemiological Studies. *Law Med Health Care* (1991):19:247–258.
9. Soskolne, C.L., and A. Light. Toward Ethics Guidelines for Environmental Epidemiologists. *Total Environ* (1996):184:137–147.
10. Last, J. Professional Standards of Conduct for Epidemiologists. In: Coughlin, S.S., and T.L. Beauchamp, editors, *Ethics and Epidemiology*. New York, NY: Oxford University Press (1996):53–75.
11. Beauchamp, T.L. Moral Foundations. In: Coughlin, S.S., and T.L. Beauchamp, editors, *Ethics and Epidemiology*. New York, NY: Oxford University Press (1996):24–52.
12. Coughlin, S.S. On the Role of Ethics Committees in Epidemiology Professional Societies. *Am J Epidemiol* (1997):146:209–213.
13. Hogue, C.J.R. Ethical Issues in Sharing Epidemiologic Data. *J Clin Epidemiol* (1991):44(I Suppl):103S–107S.

14. American College of Epidemiology. Draft Policy Statement on Privacy of Medical Records. *Epidemiol Monitor* (1998):19:9–11.

15. Clayton, E.W., K.K. Steinberg, M.J. Khoury, et al. Informed Consent for Genetic Research on Stored Tissue Samples. *JAMA* (1995):274:1786–1792.

16. Goodman, K.W., and R.J. Prineas. Toward an Ethics Curriculum in Epidemiology. In: Coughlin, S.S. and T.L. Beauchamp, editors, *Ethics and Epidemiology*. New York, NY: Oxford University Press (1996):290–303.

17. Coughlin, S.S., and G.D. Etheredge. On the Need for Ethics Curricula in Epidemiology. *Epidemiology* (1995):6:566–567.

18. Coughlin, S.S. Model Curricula in Public Health Ethics. *Am J Prev Med* (1996):12:247–251.

19. Rossignol, A.M., and S. Goodmonson. Are Ethical Topics in Epidemiology Included in the Graduate Epidemiology Curricula? *Am J Epidemiol* (1996):142:1265–1268.

20. Fayerweather, W.E., J. Higginson, and T.L. Beauchamp, editors. *Industrial Epidemiology Forum's Conference on Ethics in Epidemiology. J Clin Epidemiol* (1991):44(Suppl I)1S–169S.

21. Coughlin, S.S., editor. *Ethics in Epidemiology and Clinical Research: Annotated Readings.* Newton, MA: Epidemiology Resources, Inc. (1995).

22. Coughlin, S.S. and T.L. Beauchamp, editors. *Ethics and Epidemiology*. New York, NY: Oxford University Press (1996).

23. Soskolne, C.L., and R. Bertollini, editors. *Ethical and Philosophical Issues in Environmental Epidemiology. Proceedings of a WHO/ISEE International Workshop*, 16–18 September 1994, Research Triangle Park, NC, USA. *Sci Total Environ* (1996):184:1–147.

24. Weed, D.L. Science, Ethics Guidelines, and Advocacy in Epidemiology. *Ann Epidemiol* (1994):4:166–171.

25. Rothman, K.J., and C. Poole. Science and Policy Making (Editorial). *Am J Public Health* (1985):75:340–341.

26. Krieger, N. Questioning Epidemiology: Objectivity, Advocacy, and Socially Responsible Science. *Am J Public Health* (1999):89:1151–1156.

27. Soskolne, C.L. Epidemiological Research, Interest Groups, and the Review Process. *J Public Health Policy* (1985):7:173–184.

28. Rothman, K.J. Conflict of Interest: the New McCarthyism in Science. *JAMA* (1993):269: 2782–2784.

29. Rothman, K.J., and C.I. Cann. Judging Words Rather than Authors (Editorial). *Epidemiology* (1997):8:223–225.

30. Manson, J.E. Adventures in Scientific Discourse. *Epidemiology* (1997):8:324–326.

31. Soskolne, C.L., editor. *Proceedings of the Symposium on Ethics and Law in Environmental Epidemiology. J Exp Anal Environ Epidemiol* (1993):3(1 Suppl):243–319.

32. Soskolne, C.L., and D.K. MacFarlane. Scientific Misconduct in Epidemiologic Research. In: Coughlin, S.S., and T.L. Beauchamp, editors, *Ethics and Epidemiology*. New York, NY: Oxford University Press (1996):274–289.

33. Weed, D. L. Preventing Scientific Misconduct. *Am J Public Health* (1998):88:125–129.

34. Gellermann, W., M.S. Frankel, and R.F. Ladenson. *Values and Ethics in Organization and Human Systems Development. Responding to Dilemmas in Professional Life.* San Francisco, CA: Jossey-Bass (1990).

35. Flores, A., editor. *Professional Ideals*. Belmont, CA: Wadsworth Publication (1988).

36. Coughlin, S.S. Scientific Paradigms in Epidemiology and Professional Values. *Epidemiology* (1998):9:578–580.

37. Levy, B.S. Creating the Future of Public Health: Values, Vision, and Leadership. *Am J Public Health* (1998):88:188–192.

38. Weed, D.L. Epistemology and Ethics in Epidemiology. In: Coughlin, S.S., and T.L. Beauchamp, editors, *Ethics and Epidemiology*. New York, NY: Oxford University Press (1996): 76–94.

39. Weed, D.L., and R.E. McKeown. Epidemiology and Virtue Ethics. *Int J Epidemiol* (1998):27:343–349.

40. Pellegrino, E.D. Toward a Virtue-Based Normative Ethics for the Health Professions. *Kennedy Inst Ethics J* (1995):5:253–277.

41. Annas, G.J., and S. Elias. *Gene Mapping: Using Law and Ethics as Guides*. New York, NY: Oxford University Press (1992).

42. Faden, R., and N. Kass. HIV Research, Ethics, and the Developing World (Editorial). *Am J Public Health* (1998):88:548–550.

43. Perinatal HIV Intervention Research in Developing Countries Workshop Participants. Consensus Statement: Science, Ethics, and the Future of Research into Maternal Infant Transmission of HIV-1. *Lancet* (1999):353:832–835.

44. American College of Epidemiology. History. Available at http://www.acepidemiology.org/history.html. Accessed December 26, 1998.

45. International Society for Environmental Epidemiology. *Mission and Philosophy*. Available at http://www.iseepi.org/about/mission.html. Accessed March 15, 2000.

46. Centers for Disease Control and Prevention. *Core Values*. Available at http://www.cdc.gov/aboutcdc.htm#values. Accessed February 3, 2000.

47. National Institutes of Health. *Overview*. Available at http://www.nih.gov/about/almanac97/overview.htm. Accessed December 26, 1998.

48. UT–Houston School of Public Health. *Mission Statement*. Available at http://www.sph.uth.tmc.edu/about/default.aspx?id=65. Accessed October 1998.

49. Weed, D.L., and S.S. Coughlin. New Ethics Guidelines for Epidemiology: Background and Rationale. *Ann Epidemiol* (1999):9:277–280.

50. Council for International Organizations of Medical Sciences. *International Ethical Guidelines for Biomedical Research Involving Human Subjects*. Geneva: CIOMS (1993).

51. Declaration of Helsinki—Nothing to Declare? (Editorial). *Lancet* (1999):353:1285.

52. Soskolne, C.L., G.S. Jhangri, B. Hunter, et al. Interim Report on the Joint International Society for Environmental Epidemiology (ISEE)—Global Environmental Epidemiology Network (GEENET) Ethics Survey. *Sci Total Environ* (1996):184:5–11.

53. Prineas, R.J., K. Goodman, C.L. Soskolne, et al. Findings from the American College of Epidemiology Ethics Survey on the Need for Ethics Guidelines for Epidemiologists. *Ann Epidemiol* (1998):8:482–429.

54. Coughlin, S.S., G.D. Etheredge, C. Metayer, et al. Remember Tuskegee: Public Health Student Knowledge of the Ethical Significance of the Tuskegee Syphilis Study. *Am J Prev Med* (1996):12:242–246.

55. Coughlin, S.S., W.H. Katz, and D.R. Mattison. Ethics Instruction at Schools of Public Health in the United States. *Am J Public Health* (1999):89:768–770.

56. Committee for the Study of the Future of Public Health, Institute of Medicine. *The Future of Public Health*. Washington, D.C.: National Academies Press, 1988.

57. Krieger, N., and S. Zierler. What Explains the Public's Health? A Call for Epidemiologic Theory. *Epidemiology* (1996):7:107–109.

58. Morris, J.N. Modern Epidemiology? *J Epidemiol Community Health* (1988):42:100.

59. Terris, M. The Society for Epidemiologic Research (SER) and the Future of Epidemiology. *Am J Epidemiol* (1992):136:909–915.

60. Pearce, N. Traditional Epidemiology, Modern Epidemiology, and Public Health. *Am J Public Health* (1996):86:678–683.

61. Susser, M., and E. Susser. Choosing a Future for Epidemiology: I. Eras and Paradigms. *Am J Public Health* 1996:86:668–673.

62. Susser, M., and E. Susser. Choosing a Future for Epidemiology: II. From Black Box to Chinese Boxes and Eco-Epidemiology. *Am J Public Health* (1996):86:674–677.

63. Last, J.M. What Is "Clinical Epidemiology?" *J Public Health Policy* (1988):9:159–163.

64. Gori, G.B. Epidemiology and Public Health: Is a New Paradigm Needed for a New Ethic? *J Clin Epidemiol* (1998):51:637–641.

65. Weed, D.L. Beyond Black Box Epidemiology. *Am J Public Health* (1998):88:12–14.

66. Pearce, N., and J.B. McKinlay. Back to the Future in Epidemiology and Public Health: Response to Dr. Gori. *J Clin Epidemiol* (1998):51:643–646.

67. Coughlin, S.S., C.L. Soskolne, and K.W. Goodman. *Case Studies in Public Health Ethics.* Washington, D.C.: American Public Health Association (1997).

68. Bloom, S.W. Reform without Change? Look Beyond the Curriculum (Editorial). *Am J Public Health* (1995):907–908.

69. Hunter, D., and N. Caporaso. Informed Consent in Epidemiologic Studies Involving Genetic Markers. *Epidemiology* (1997):8:596–599.

70. DHHS Preparing to Promulgate Privacy Regulation if Congress Fails to Pass New Privacy Law. *Epidemiology Monitor* (1999):20:7–8.

71. Campbell, S.G., G.L. Gibby, and S. Collingwood. The Internet and Electronic Transmission of Medical Records. *J Clin Monitoring* (1997):13:325–334.

72. Barrows, R.C., and P.D. Clayton. Privacy, Confidentiality, and Electronic Medical Records. *J Am Med Inform Assoc* (1996):3:139–148.

73. Coughlin, S.S. Ethics in Epidemiology and Public Health Practice. In: Coughlin, S.S., editor, *Epidemiology and Public Health Practice: Collected Works.* Columbus, GA: Quill Publications (1997):9–26.

74. Soskolne, C.L. Rationalizing Professional Conduct: Ethics in Disease Control. *Public Health Rev* (1991):19:311–321.

75. Wartenberg, D. Ethics in Community-Based Environmental Epidemiology and Public Health Practice: Some Considerations. *Sci Total Environ* 1996:184:109–112.

CHAPTER 2

ETHICS IN EPIDEMIOLOGY: COMMON MISCONCEPTIONS, PARADOXES, AND UNRESOLVED QUESTIONS

Steven S. Coughlin

Important advances occurred in ethics and epidemiology in the past few decades as highlighted in several reviews [1–4]. These advances include the development and refinement of ethics guidelines and standards of conduct for epidemiologists [5–9], the formulation of policy statements and committee reports on such topics as data sharing, privacy and confidentiality protection, and genetic testing for disease susceptibility [10–12], the development of ethics curricula in epidemiology and public health [13–18], and a burgeoning international literature on ethical and social issues in epidemiology [19–38]. Ethics case studies, with discussion questions suitable for use in the classroom or in continuing education programs for epidemiologists, have also been published and incorporated into CD-ROM educational resources [39].

Previous articles have listed specific issues and controversies in ethics and epidemiology, and proposed organizational frameworks for thinking and communication about important developments in this area. Goodman and Prineas [14] enumerated what they considered to be the core components of a course in ethics and epidemiology (consideration of moral foundations; duties, responsibilities, and practice standards; valid consent and refusal; risks, harms, and wrongs; sponsorship and conflict of interests; communications, publication, intellectual property, and education; advocacy and intercultural conflict). Soskolne and Sieswerda [29] proposed a framework for implementing ethics in environmental epidemiology and related professions, which they divided into foundations (professional organization and statement of core values) and implementation (ethics guidelines; organizational infrastructure and established procedures; ethics education and training; ethics consultation service; and ongoing oversight and commitment). Such lists and frameworks have often included important milestones, such as the development of ethics guidelines for epidemiologists, and questions that are as yet unresolved, or only partially clarified (e.g., some issues surrounding conflicts of interest and the publication of research findings) [40–43]. Some of the key issues that have been highlighted in prior contributions represent ethical disputes, or ongoing controversies. Others relate to what I believe to be misconceptions commonly held by epidemiologists, or members of stakeholder groups. In this paper, I identify and comment on unresolved questions and key issues, with the goal of clarifying and generating further support for professional ethics in epidemiology.

"Ethics in Epidemiology: Common Misconceptions, Paradoxes, and Unresolved Questions" originally appeared in the Journal of Epidemiology and Biostatistics (2000):5:25–29. Used with permission of Taylor and Francis. http://www.informaworld.com

Common Misconceptions

One common misconception (in my experience) is that ethics in epidemiology primarily has to do with the correction of ethical lapses, or the identification and "punishment" of "wrongdoers." Media coverage of high-visibility cases of alleged scientific misconduct and exposés on human subjects' concerns may have contributed to this impression. In fact, much of the emphasis in ethics in epidemiology is instead on the clarification of a variety of professional duties and on ethical norms and precepts that are still evolving. These include ethical issues about which reasonable persons may be apt to disagree. Examples include optimal rules or guidelines for the sharing of epidemiologic data, how best to communicate epidemiologic research findings, and the extent to which epidemiologists should engage in public health advocacy [10, 32, 44–46]. Nevertheless, high visibility cases and controversies can lead to the clarification of ethical duties of health researchers and to renewed attention on the broader social consequences of health research [25, 47, 48]. Examples include the ethics of vaccine trials, research carried out in the developing world by investigators from developed countries, public concern over the scientific integrity of health research, and ethical issues in genetics research [12, 47–53].

Another misconception is that difficult ethical issues in epidemiology are best left to experts, such as trained bioethicists and legal scholars. Although input from scholars in other disciplines is important, it is equally important that practicing epidemiologists contribute to the identification and clarification of ethical issues and controversies. Few bioethicists and legal experts are familiar with the concepts and terminology of epidemiology, and relatively few persons outside of public health are intimately familiar with core values and ethical norms in epidemiology and public health. Exceptions to these general statements can be cited, however, including individuals who have made important contributions to the literature on public health ethics.

Epidemiologists contribute to the resolution of ethical disputes and advance our understanding of ethical precepts, by discussing ethical issues at professional meetings, at workshops, in the classroom, and in public forums, and by publishing articles and letters to the editor. The ideal situation is for both epidemiologists and scholars from such fields as bioethics and health law to contribute to ongoing discussions about ethics and epidemiology, while interacting and communicating with each other. This will require epidemiologists to become better acquainted with key ethics concepts and nomenclature and, conversely, for interested scholars from other disciplines to become acquainted with epidemiologic concepts and terminology. Although an increasing number of epidemiologists have become well versed in bioethics, and epidemiologists from several countries have contributed to the ethics literature, there is a need to ensure that junior epidemiologists and students enrolled in graduate training programs become engaged in ethics discussions. Furthering professional ethics in epidemiology requires thoughtful discussion and an understanding of the underlying ethical principles.

Another misconception that I have found to be common among both epidemiologists and bioethicists is that ethics cases and ethical dilemmas in public health are less important or compelling from a human-interest standpoint than those in other areas of biomedical research ethics and clinical ethics (e.g., bioethics cases related to organ transplantation, the use of artificial organs, human cloning, maternal–fetal conflict, or difficult decisions that must be made at the end of life) [54, 55]. There are many ethical dilemmas and ethics cases in public health that are equally compelling from the standpoint of both human interest and social importance. For example, gripping narrative stories and ethics cases have emerged from epidemiologic responses to the AIDS pandemic, interpersonal violence, homelessness, perinatal health concerns, issues surrounding the maldistribution of health care resources, and occupational and environmental health concerns [24, 39, 56–61]. However, not all are published, or readily accessible to interested readers. Others are written for a specialized audience in the detached, scientific tone that characterizes the bulk of the scientific literature, rather than being emotionally charged, or written in a discursive manner. Areas in which further published ethics cases are needed include field epidemiology, public health surveillance of communicable diseases, and other important topics in public health practice [24, 39, 62, 63].

A fourth misconception that, hopefully, is becoming less common, is that by deepening our attention to ethical concerns in epidemiology (e.g., by calling for updated ethics guidelines or formal training in ethics for epidemiology graduate students and practicing epidemiologists), we are somehow making the lives of epidemiologists more difficult or potentially creating encumbrances. Steps taken to strengthen professional ethics in epidemiology—including measures that safeguard scientific integrity and protect the rights and welfare of research participants—actually help to maintain public trust and generate support for the work that epidemiologists perform [3, 30]. Epidemiologists should contribute to discussions about how best to protect the rights and welfare of research participants and the general public, while facilitating epidemiologic studies. Public trust is essential if epidemiologic activities are to continue to be supported by the public and by funding sources. Ethical analyses and position papers on such diverse topics as the privacy and confidentiality of medical records, institutional review board procedures in the United States, and genetics research involving the use of biological specimens, have indirectly helped maintain research opportunities for epidemiologists and furthered the public interest [11, 12, 64].

Ethical Paradoxes in Epidemiology and Other Areas of Health Research

Simply defined, a paradox is a statement that seems to conflict with common sense, or to contradict itself, but that may nevertheless be true [65]. One paradoxical observation is that unfortunate or even disastrous episodes in human subjects research can have desirable consequences in addition to the undesirable (or extraordinarily undesirable) consequences with which they have been associated. This observation provides an argument both for strengthening efforts to prevent recurrences of such problems and for reflecting on the important lessons of historical cases [17]. To cite one example from public health, the Tuskegee Syphilis Study, which has become a metaphor for racism in medicine and ethical misconduct in human subjects research, was one of the historical events that led to improved federal regulations in the United States for the protection of human subjects [17, 66–68]. Lasting concern over the legacy of the Tuskegee Syphilis Study has been a stimulus for more recent efforts to strengthen researchers' training in bioethics [68]. Although such historical events have, fortunately, been rare and will, hopefully, not occur in the future, there is an ongoing need to remember the lessons of the past, and to take steps to maintain and restore public confidence in public health institutions. This is especially true among minority communities, such as African Americans. Paradigmatic cases in public health ethics, such as the Tuskegee Syphilis Study, are an important part of professional education on ethics that should be included in graduate training and continuing education programs for epidemiologists [15, 17].

Another seemingly paradoxical observation is that measures taken to protect potential research participants from risks and harms can have unexpected, undesirable consequences. For example, in response to public concern over the thalidomide disaster and other developments that had occurred by the 1960s, new regulations were adopted in the United States and other countries that provided added protections for participants in clinical investigations [4, 69]. There was focused concern over the rights and welfare of vulnerable groups (or groups that were perceived to be vulnerable), such as women of childbearing ages, children, the elderly, persons with diminished mental capacity, and institutionalized persons [70]. Some of the regulatory safeguards and institutional policies adopted at that time had the undesirable effect of excluding women and children from clinical trials of experimental therapies, which led to a paucity of evidence about which treatments were safe and effective among those population subgroups. In recent years, there has been increased emphasis on ensuring that women, children, and other population subgroups (e.g., minorities and the elderly) have access to clinical studies that may provide beneficial information [71, 72]. The same is true of public health research, including epidemiologic studies.

Unresolved Questions

Some scientific questions in epidemiology cannot be answered using widely accepted research methods because of ethical constraints. For example, it would not be ethically acceptable to undertake a randomized controlled trial of cigarette smoking and risk of various disease outcomes in human volunteers. Constraints due to ethical and social concerns may also arise in observational studies. For example, in some cultures, questions about some aspects of human sexuality or reproduction are too sensitive to be directly addressed in research questionnaires. However, ethical and social constraints on epidemiologic research do not necessarily preclude the acquisition of important scientific information, through which public health problems can be addressed. For example, results obtained from case-control and cohort studies and other lines of evidence (including results from laboratory experiments and animal studies) showed that cigarette smoking is a cause of lung cancer.

Are there any *ethical* questions in epidemiology that are unanswerable with present methods and theoretical frameworks, or because of constraints from other ethical concerns? One set of questions relates to the ethical knowledge, attitudes, and practices of epidemiologists, as well as their ethical decision-making skills. Information about the ethics knowledge and attitudes of epidemiologists and students enrolled in epidemiology graduate courses has been obtained through survey research [13, 16, 17, 73]. Studies to date have not assessed the ability of epidemiologists or epidemiology students to identify and resolve ethical dilemmas through ethical reasoning, or their ability to evaluate ethical problems in public health. Nevertheless, studies of medical residents and students enrolled in medical and dental schools have addressed such questions using "paper and pencil" tests of moral-reasoning ability developed for health professionals [74, 75]. Some data also exist about the prevalence of scientific misconduct in scientific fields (but not epidemiology, in particular) [47, 48]. This should not be surprising since researchers have learned how to collect sensitive information from research participants about socially undesirable or illicit behaviors in ways that ensure that the responses are reasonably reliable and valid, and which protect the respondents from risks and potential harms, such as those posed by breaches of confidentiality. Although some questions about the ethical knowledge, attitudes, practices, and decision-making skills of epidemiologists may be difficult to clarify, we have not reached the limits of what could be clarified with current methods and theoretical frameworks for understanding professional ethics.

What about questions relating to the ethical duties of epidemiologists, or the broader social consequences of epidemiologic research? Such questions have been addressed in considerable detail in ethics guidelines for epidemiologists and in the broader literature on ethics in epidemiology. Nevertheless, a consensus is presently lacking about some ethical questions in epidemiology. In addition, new ethical concerns and dilemmas will continue to arise in epidemiology, as new research methods and technologies are developed and as new public health concerns arise. Available approaches for learning more and building a consensus include incisive analyses by epidemiologists, bioethicists, and legal scholars; further research on ethics and sociopolitical issues in the field by epidemiologists, historians, sociologists, political scientists, and scholars in African-American studies and women's studies; and exploring the significance and meaning of epidemiology's role in society through the humanities, including literature, art, theater, and the history of public health [76].

Some ethical questions in epidemiology remain only partly answered, or they relate to ethical precepts that are still evolving. In addition to examples cited elsewhere in this paper, these include ethical issues surrounding the role of lay epidemiologists in environmental health studies; how best to avoid the stigmatization of communities that are targeted by epidemiologic studies while at the same time disseminating important information that may provide benefits to those same communities; and certain additional issues that arise in community surveys and cross-cultural research [8, 24, 28]. Nevertheless, substantial progress has been made in recent years in such areas as disclosure of information and avoidance of risks and potential harm in genetics research; clarification of ethical duties and obligations in AIDS research; obtaining informed consent in cross-cultural studies; and how best to balance concerns about the privacy and confidentiality of health information with public health objectives.

Some important ethical questions in epidemiology may be unanswered at present (e.g., some human subjects issues surrounding the inclusion of undocumented workers and illegal immigrants in health studies carried out in the United States and European countries) and others may even be unanswerable. Nevertheless, the many accomplishments achieved in ethics and epidemiology in the closing decade of the twentieth century indicate there is good reason to be optimistic that more achievements in this area lie ahead and that this will translate into sustained support for the important work that epidemiologists perform in the public interest.

Acknowledgments

The author is grateful to John Last and Colin Soskolne for their helpful comments on an earlier draft of this manuscript.

References

1. Soskolne, C.L. Epidemiology: Questions of Science, Ethics, Morality, and Law. *Am J Epidemiol* (1989):129:1–18.
2. Last, J. Professional Standards of Conduct for Epidemiologists. In: Coughlin, S.S., and T.L. Beauchamp, editors, *Ethics and Epidemiology*. New York, NY: Oxford University Press (1996):53–75.

3. Coughlin, S.S. Advancing Professional Ethics in Epidemiology. *J Epidemiol Biostat* (1996):1:71–77.
4. Coughlin, S.S., and T.L. Beauchamp. Historical Foundations. In: Coughlin, S.S., and T.L. Beauchamp, editors, *Ethics and Epidemiology*. New York: Oxford University Press (1996):5–23.
5. International Epidemiological Association. Ethical Guidelines for Epidemiologists (draft). *Epidemiology Section Newsletter* (1990) Winter.
6. Beauchamp, T.L., R.R. Cook, W.E. Fayerweather, et al. Ethical Guidelines for Epidemiologists. *J Clin Epidemiol* (1991):44:151S–169S.
7. Council for International Organizations of Medical Sciences. International Guidelines for Ethical Review of Epidemiological Studies. *Law Med Health Care* (1991):19:247–258.
8. Soskolne, C.L., and A. Light. Toward Ethics Guidelines for Environmental Epidemiologists. *Total Environ* (1996):184:137–147.
9. Weed, D.L., and S.S. Coughlin. New Ethics Guidelines for Epidemiologists. *Total Environ* (1996):184:137–147.
10. Hogue, C.J.R. Ethical Issues in Sharing Epidemiologic Data. *J Clin Epidemiol* (1991):44(I Suppl):103S–107S.
11. American College of Epidemiology. Draft Policy Statement on Privacy of Medical Records. *Epidemiol Monitor* (1998):19:9–11.
12. Clayton, E.W., K.K. Steinberg, M.J. Khoury, et al. Informed Consent for Genetic Research on Stored Tissue Samples. *J Am Med Assoc* (1995):274:1786–1792.
13. Coughlin, S.S., and G.D. Etheredge. On the Need for Ethics Curricula in Epidemiology. *Epidemiology* (1995):6:566–567.
14. Goodman, K.W., and R.J. Prineas. Toward an Ethics Curriculum in Epidemiology. In: Coughlin, S.S., and T.L. Beauchamp, editors, *Ethics and Epidemiology*. New York, NY: Oxford University Press (1996):290–303.
15. Coughlin, S.S. Model Curricula in Public Health Ethics. *Am J Prev Med* (1996):12: 247–251.
16. Rossignol, A.M., and S. Goodmonson. Are Ethical Topics in Epidemiology Included in the Graduate Epidemiology Curricula. *Am J Epidemiol* (1996):142:1265–1268.
17. Coughlin, S.S., G.D. Etheredge, C. Metayer, et al. Remember Tuskegee: Public Health Student Knowledge of the Ethical Significance of the Tuskegee Syphilis Study. *Am J Prev Med* (1996):12:242–246.
18. Coughlin, S.S., W.H. Katz, and D.R. Mattison. Ethics Instruction at Schools of Public Health in the United States. *Am J Public Health* (1999):89:768–770.
19. Gordis, L., E. Gold, and R. Seltser. Privacy Protection in Epidemiologic and Medical Research: A Challenge and a Responsibility. *Am J Epidemiol* (1977):105:163–168.
20. Susser, M., Z. Stein, and J. Kline. Ethics in Epidemiology. *Ann Am Acad Polit Soc Sci* (1978): 437:128–141.
21. Weed, D.L., and R.E. McKeown. Epidemiology and Virtue Ethics. *Int J Epidemiol* (1998): 27:343–349.
22. Prineas, R.J., K. Goodman, C.L. Soskolne, et al. Findings from the American College of Epidemiology Ethics Survey on the Need for Ethics Guidelines for Epidemiologists. *Ann Epidemiol* (1998):8:482–489.
23. Hunter, D., and N. Caporaso. Informed Consent in Epidemiologic Studies Involving Genetic Markers. *Epidemiology* (1997):8:596–599.
24. Coughlin, S.S. *Epidemiologic and Public Health Practice: Collected Works*. Columbus, GA: Quill Publications (1997):9–26.
25. Soskolne, C.L., editor. Proceedings of the Symposium on Ethics and Law in Environmental Epidemiology. *J Exp Anal Environ Epidemiol* (1993):3(1 Suppl):243–319.
26. Fayerweather, W.E., J. Higginson, and T.L. Beauchamp, editors. Industrial Epidemiology Forum's Conference on Ethics in Epidemiology. *J Clin Epidemiol* (1991):44(I Suppl).

27. Coughlin, S.S., editor. *Ethics in Epidemiology and Clinical Research: Annotated Readings.* Newton, MA: Epidemiology Resources (1995).

28. Coughlin, S.S., and T.L. Beauchamp, editors. *Ethics and Epidemiology.* New York, NY: Oxford University Press (1996).

29. Soskolne, C.L., and L.E. Sieswerda. Implementing Ethics in the Professions: Toward Ecological Integrity. *Ecosystem Health* (1998):4:109–118.

30. Coughlin, S.S. On the Role of Ethics Committees in Epidemiology Professional Societies. *Am J Epidemiol* (1997):146:209–113.

31. Soskolne, C.L., and R. Bertollini, editors. Ethical and Philosophical Issues in Environmental Epidemiology. *Proceedings of a WHO/ISEE International Workshop,* 16–18 September 1994, Research Triangle Park, NC, USA. *Science Total Environ* (1996):184.

32. Weed, D.L. Science, Ethics Guidelines, and Advocacy in Epidemiology. *Ann Epidemiol* (1994): 4:166–171.

33. Soskolne, C.L. Epidemiological Research, Interest Groups, and the Review Process. *J Public Health Policy* (1985):7:173–184.

34. Benecko, V. Modern Ethical Problems in Environmental Epidemiology. [Czech] *Epidemiol Microbiol Immunol* (1995):44:180–183.

35. Last, J. New pathways in an age of ecological and ethical concerns. *Int J Epidemiol* (1994):23:1–4.

36. Horner, J.S. Research, Ethics, and Privacy: the Limits of Knowledge. *Publ Health* (1998): 112:217–220.

37. Comba, P. The Ethical Problem of the Health–Environment Relationship. [Italian]. *Ann Ist Super Sanità* (1997):33:279–284.

38. Khan, K.S. Epidemiology and Ethics: the Perspective of the Third World. *J Public Health Policy* (1994):15:218–225.

39. Coughlin, S.S., C.L. Soskolne, and K.W. Goodman. *Case Studies in Public Health Ethics.* Washington, D.C.: American Public Health Association (1997).

40. Rothman, K.J. Conflict of Interest: the New McCarthyism in Science. *J Am Med Assoc* (1993):269:2782–2784.

41. Rothman, K.J., and C.I. Cann. Judging Words Rather than Authors (Editorial). *Epidemiology* (1997):8:223–225.

42. Manson, J.E. Adventures in Scientific Discourse. *Epidemiology* (1997):8:324–326.

43. Szklo, M. Issues in Publication and Interpretation of Research Findings. *J Clin Epidemiol* (1991):44:109S–113S.

44. Rothman, K.J., and C. Poole. Science and Policy Making [Editorial]. *Am J Public Health* (1985):75:340–341.

45. Sandman, P.M. Emerging Communication Responsibilities of Epidemiologists. *J Clin Epidemiol* (1991):44(I Suppl)41S–50S.

46. Schulte, P.A. Ethical Issues in the Communication of Results. *J Clin Epidemiol* (1991):44(I Suppl):57S–61S.

47. Soskolne, C.L., and D.K. MacFarlane. Scientific Misconduct in Epidemiologic Research. In: Coughlin, S.S., and T.L. Beauchamp, editors, *Ethics and Epidemiology.* New York, NY: Oxford University Press (1996):274–89.

48. Weed, D.L. Preventing Scientific Misconduct. *Am J Public Health* (1998):88:125–129.

49. Annas, G.J., and S. Elias. *Gene Mapping: Using Law and Ethics as Guides.* New York, NY: Oxford University Press (1992).

50. Angell, M. Ethical Imperialism? Ethics in International Collaborative Clinical Research (Editorial). *N Engl J Med* (1988):319:1081–1083.

51. Ijsselmuiden, C.B., and R.R. Faden. Research and Informed Consent in Africa—Another Look. *N Engl J Med* (1992):326:830–834.

52. Mariner, W.K. Why Clinical Trials of AIDS Vaccines Are Premature. *Publ Health Law* (1989): 79:86–91.

53. Christakis, NA. The Ethical Design of an AIDS Vaccine Trial in Africa. *Hastings Center Rep* (1988):18:31–37.

54. Annas, G.J. *Standard of Care. The Law of American Bioethics.* New York, NY: Oxford University Press (1993).

55. Veatch, R.M. *Case Studies in Medical Ethics.* Cambridge, MA: Harvard University Press (1977).

56. Reamer, F.G., editor. *AIDS and Ethics.* New York, NY: Columbia University Press (1991).

57. Oppenheimer, G.M. In the Eye of the Storm: the Epidemiological Construction of AIDS. In: Fee, E., and D.M. Fox, editors, *AIDS: the Burdens of History.* Berkeley, CA: University of California Press (1988):267–300.

58. Mann, J.M., D.J.M. Tarantola, and T.W. Netter, editors. *AIDS in the World.* Cambridge, MA: Harvard University Press (1992).

59. McCord, C., and H.P. Freeman. Excess Mortality in Harlem. *N Engl J Med* (1990):332: 173–177.

60. Link, B.G., E. Susser, A. Stueve, et al. Lifetime and Five-Year Prevalence of Homelessness in the United States. *Am J Public Health* (1994):84:1907–1912.

61. Proctor, R.N. Cancer Wars. How Politics Shapes What We Know and Don't Know about Cancer. New York, NY: Basic Books (1995).

62. Soskolne, C.L. Rationalizing Professional Conduct: Ethics in Disease Control. *Public Health Rev* (1991):19:311–321.

63. Last, J.M. Ethics and Public Health Policy. In: *Public Health and Human Ecology.* Stamford, CT: Appleton and Lange (1998).

64. Cann, C.I., and K.J. Rothman. IRBs and Epidemiologic Research: How Inappropriate Restrictions Hamper Studies. *IRB* (1984):6:5–7.

65. *Webster's II New Riverside Dictionary.* New York, NY: Berkeley Books (1984).

66. Gamble, V.N. The Tuskegee Syphilis Study and Women's Health. *J Am Med Assoc* (1997): 52:195–196.

67. Jones, J.H. *Bad Blood.* New York, NY: Free Press (1993).

68. Love, C.B., E.J. Thomson, and D. Charmaine, compilers. *Ethical Issues in Research Involving Human Participants* [bibliography on the Internet]. Bethesda, MD: National Library of Medicine (1999). (*Curr Bibliog Med* 99-3). Available at http://www.nlm.nih.gov/pubs/resources.html.

69. Blake, J., editor. *Safeguarding the Public: Historical Aspects of Medicinal Drug Control.* Baltimore, MA: The Johns Hopkins University Press (1970).

70. National Commission for the Protection of Human Subjects of Biomedical and Behavioral Research. *The Belmont Report: Ethical Principles and Guidelines for the Protection of Human Subjects of Research.* Washington, D.C.: US Government Printing Office (1978).

71. Kinney, E.L., J. Trautmann, J.A. Gold, et al. Underrepresentation of Women in New Drug Trials. *Ann Intern Med* (1981):95:495–499.

72. Mastroianni, A.C., R. Faden, and D. Federman, editors, *Women and Health Research. Ethical and Legal Issues of Including Women in Clinical Studies,* vol. I. Washington, D.C.: National Academies Press (1994).

73. Soskolne, C.L., G.S. Jhangri, B. Hunter, et al. Interim Report on the Joint International Society for Environmental Epidemiology (ISEE)—Global Environmental Epidemiology Network (GEENET) Ethics Survey. *Sci Total Environ* (1996):184:5–11.

74. Self, D.J., and J.D. Skeel. Facilitating Health Care Ethics Research: Assessment of Moral Reasoning and Moral Orientation from a Single Interview. *Camb Q Healthc Ethics* (1992):4: 371–376.

75. Bebeau, M.J., J.R. Rest, and C.M. Yamoor. Measuring Dental Students' Ethical Sensitivity. *J Dent Educ* (1985):49:225–235.

76. Weed, D.L. Epidemiology, Humanities, and Public Health. *Am J Public Health* (1995):85:914–918.

PART II

FOUNDATIONAL ISSUES PERTAINING TO ETHICS IN EPIDEMIOLOGY AND PUBLIC HEALTH

Public health ethics, which can be defined as the identification, analysis, and resolution of ethical problems arising in public health practice and research, has different domains from those of medical ethics, organizational ethics, or professional ethics. Childress et al. [1] have noted that public health ethics includes a loose set of general moral considerations (values, principles, or rules) that are relevant to public health. The focus in public health ethics is on identifying, weighing, and balancing the ethical values and moral claims at stake in a particular public health decision (e.g., deciding how best to distribute scarce resources during a pandemic, whether to mandate the wearing of bicycle helmets, or whether to quarantine someone with an infectious strain of tuberculosis). Proposed analytic frameworks for health policy and program planning have often considered the goals of a program, its effectiveness, known or potential burdens, the balance of burdens and potential benefits, and fairness in implementation (e.g., the distributional consequences of a public health intervention). Deliberations about the fairness of public health interventions and how they are implemented are informed by the broader literature on equity in health (including how best to measure health inequalities) and theories of justice [2, 3]. Least restrictive infringement, public justification, transparency, and proportionality of benefits and burdens have also been cited as important considerations for health policy and program planning.

The article included in this section provides an overview of principle-based methods of moral reasoning as they apply to public health ethics, including a summary of advantages and disadvantages of methods of moral reasoning that rely on general principles of moral reasoning. Examples are provided of additional principles, obligations, and rules that may be useful for analyzing complex ethical issues in public health. A framework is outlined that takes into consideration the interplay of ethical principles and rules at different levels (e.g., at the individual, community, and national levels, or globally). As noted in the article, different accounts of ethics may point to different principles. Public health ethics does not entail a commitment to any particular philosophic or ethical theory, nor do various frameworks proposed in the literature on ethics in epidemiology and public health practice necessarily point to the same sets of moral principles and values. The resulting complexity is increased by the tendency of philosophers to use the term "principle" to refer to widely varied concepts. This includes principles of solidarity and social cohesion and the precautionary principle that have frequently been cited in public health and the environmental sciences.

As noted in the following article, the *precautionary principle* asserts that when an activity threatens harm to human health or the environment, precautionary measures should be taken even if some cause-and-effect relationships are not fully established. In public health practice and environmental protection, there is frequently a need to take preventive action even in the face of scientific uncertainty. Critics have charged that the precautionary principle focuses on hypothetical risks rather than actual hazards and that other analytic methods (e.g., cost-effectiveness and cost-benefit analyses) may provide a more suitable basis for regulation. A further issue is that, in the face of limited resources for prevention activities, putting resources into untested or ineffective interventions (e.g., the use of intervention approaches that are not evidence-based and which have not been shown to be effective in rigorous studies) may result in the withholding of resources from other activities that are more effective. This illustrates that theoretical discussions about proposed analytic frameworks for ethical decision-making, health policymaking, program planning, and the setting of prevention priorities can have important implications for public health.

1. Childress, J.F., R.R. Faden, R.D. Gaare, et al. Public Health Ethics: Mapping the Terrain. *J Law Med Ethics* (2002):30:170–178.
2. Anand, S., F. Peter, and A. Sen. *Public Health, Ethics, and Equity.* New York, NY: Oxford University Press (2004).
3. Powers, M., and R. Faden. *Social Justice: The Moral Foundations of Public Health and Health Policy.* New York, NY: Oxford University Press (2008).

CHAPTER 3

HOW MANY PRINCIPLES FOR PUBLIC HEALTH ETHICS?

Steven S. Coughlin

The words "principle" and "principles" have several different meanings in moral philosophy, science, and common usage. Principles are sometimes taken to be basic truths, laws, or assumptions, as in "the principles of democratic societies." In everyday English, a principle is a rule of personal conduct or standard of good behavior (as in, "she is a woman of principle who will not violate her principles"). In moral philosophy, principles have more to do with the ethics, value system, or moral code that is accepted by society. In many accounts, principles are seen as basic qualities that determine intrinsic nature or characteristic behavior.

General moral (ethical) principles play a prominent role in certain methods of moral reasoning and ethical decision-making in bioethics and public health [1–3]. Examples include the principles of respect for autonomy, beneficence, nonmaleficence, and justice. Although this article may strike some readers as being relatively theoretical, there have been numerous publications on ethical issues in public health practice that included more applied and less abstract discussions of important public health ethics topics (see, e.g., [4–7]). It is essential that public health professionals contribute to the identification and clarification of the ethical and moral philosophic underpinnings of their discipline, analogous to theoretical work done by leading epidemiologists to clarify causal inference in observational research [8–10].

Principles such as justice are sometimes referred to as midlevel moral principles to distinguish them from philosophical theories. Principles serve at a middle level between fundamental theory and particular rules; the latter are more restricted in scope than principles and apply to specific contexts [11]. The above list of principles is not necessarily exhaustive (e.g., principles of fidelity and veracity have been added to some accounts of bioethics [12]). In addition, some accounts of ethics in public health have pointed to additional principles related to social and environmental concerns, such as the precautionary principle and principles of solidarity or social cohesion [13, 14]. The complexity that exists because different accounts point to different principles is increased by the tendency of philosophers to use the term "principle" to refer to widely varied concepts.

This article provides an overview of principle-based methods of moral reasoning as they apply to public health ethics including a summary of advantages and disadvantages of methods of moral reasoning that rely on general principles of moral reasoning. Drawing upon the literature on public health ethics [5–7, 14–18], examples are then provided of additional principles, obligations, and rules that may be useful for analyzing complex

"How Many Principles for Public Health Ethics?" originally appeared in The Open Journal of Public Health (2008):1:8–16. Used with permission. http://bentham.org/open/tophj/index.htm

ethical issues in public health. A framework is outlined that takes into consideration the interplay of ethical principles and rules at individual, community, national, and global levels. For the sake of brevity, however, this article does not provide a full discussion of concepts of moral relativism [11, 19] or social constructionism [20, 21]. The latter refers to sociological and psychological theories of knowledge that consider how social phenomena are tied to particular social contexts.

General Moral Principles

Philosophers and bioethicists have frequently conceptualized the moral life in terms of one or more principles, although conceptualizations of moral principles have varied remarkably. In the eighteenth century, the Scottish empiricist philosopher David Hume (1711–1776) pointed to approaches to moral philosophy that sought to further our understanding of human nature by finding "those principles, which regulate our understanding, excite our sentiments, and make us approve or blame any particular object, action, or behavior." Hume noted that such philosophic approaches seek to discover truths ("ultimate principles") that will "fix, beyond controversy, the foundations of morals, reasoning, and criticism" [22]. Rather than focusing on ultimate principles, which he argued go beyond anything that can be experienced, Hume called for the establishment of an empirical approach to understanding human nature that would concentrate on describing principles that govern human nature [23]. The principles proposed by Hume (e.g., principles that attempted to account for the origins and associations of ideas) are more directly tied to human experience and perceptions than those proposed by rationalists and other philosophers. The dispute between empiricism and rationalism takes place within epistemology, the branch of philosophy devoted to studying the nature, sources, and limits of knowledge [24].

A topic central to moral reasoning is the question of what moral truths there are, if any [25]. Important questions arise from striving to provide a metaphysical grounding for moral truths and to identify what makes them true [25]. This includes questions about moral relativism and moral skepticism. Numerous philosophers have inquired, are there any true general principles of morality and, if so, what are they?

Some moral philosophers have argued that there are no defensible moral principles, and that moral reasoning does not consist of the application of moral principles to cases [26]. From this perspective, moral reasons or well-grounded moral facts can exist independently from any general principle [25]. Others have noted that, although there may be some moral principles, moral judgment requires far more than a grasp on a range of principles and the ability to apply them. In contrast to such positions, other philosophers argue that moral judgment and thought depend on the provision of suitable moral principles [26]. This contrary view holds that moral reasons are necessarily general, perhaps because a moral claim is weak if it is based solely on particularities [25]. Even if it can be established that one or more general principles are essential to moral reasoning, this leaves open the questions of whether exception-less principles are also essential to moral reasoning, and how to resolve conflicts between principles if more than one principle is accepted [25]. Moral disagreements often stem from divergent beliefs about what is morally salient and what should be counted as a moral principle [25]. John Stuart Mill (1806–1873), Immanuel Kant (1724–1804), and other philosophers from diverse schools argued that unless two options are deliberatively commensurable, it is impossible to choose rationally between them. Thus, philosophers have often sought a single, ultimate principle that could be used to resolve conflict between different moral or practical considerations.

Dancy [26] noted that there are at least two different conceptions of what moral principles are. One conception, the "absolute" conception, holds that a moral principle is a universal claim to the effect that all actions of a certain type are wrong (or right). An example of an absolute moral principle is the principle of utility in utilitarian theories, summarized below. As Dancy [26] put it, "Absolute principles, which specify a feature or combination of features that always succeed in making an action wrong (or right) wherever they occur, purport to specify an invariant overall reason . . . ." With the possible exception of theories, such as utilitarianism, in which only one principle is defended, the notion of absolute midlevel principles that must not conflict seems inconsistent with the moral life. An alternative conception views moral principles as "contributory" rather than as absolute. This contributory conception of moral principles holds that more than one principle can apply to a particular case [26]. A classic example of a moral philosophic theory based on contributory principles is W.D. Ross's [27] theory of *prima facie* duties. Ross described each *prima facie* duty as a "parti-resultant" attribute, obtained by looking at one morally relevant aspect of an act, and being one's actual duty as a "toti-resultant" attribute, obtained by looking at all of the relevant aspects [25]. Obligations cited by Ross include fidelity (which includes promise keeping and veracity), reparation, gratitude, self-improvement, justice, beneficence, and nonmaleficence (as defined below). He did not identify any general rules for estimating the comparative stringency of *prima facie* obligations, but rather pointed to the need for practical judgment. Ross [27] viewed the *prima facie* obligation of nonmaleficence as having priority over other duties such as beneficence.

The plurality of methods existing in philosophic ethics for moral reasoning includes Kantian (deontological) approaches, act and rule utilitarianism, principle-based approaches such as the principle-based common morality theory developed by Tom Beauchamp and James Childress for moral reasoning in bioethics, and many other approaches. These deductivist and nondeductivist approaches are described below, with an eye toward identifying and clarifying general moral principles in public health.

Deductivist Theories of Moral Reasoning

Moral reasoning involves deliberating about ethical questions and reaching a decision with the help of judgment and rational analysis. In such deliberations, particular decisions and actions may be justified by ethical theory (an integrated body of rules and principles). Deductivism, a common approach to justification of moral judgments and ethical decisions, involves justifying a particular judgment or belief by bringing it under one or more principles. In some cases, principles or rules are defended by a full ethical theory [11]. Two deductivist theories have commonly been cited: deontological and utilitarian [28], although these are by no means the only philosophical theories of moral reasoning that have been proposed.

Deontological theories (sometimes referred to as Kantian theories) hold that people should not be treated as means to an end and that some actions are right or wrong regardless of the consequences [11]. Kant, who viewed morality as grounded in pure reason rather than in intuition, conscience, or tradition, argued that the moral worth of an individual's action depends on the moral acceptability of the rule on which the person acts [29]. Throughout Kant's writings, "he insists that we cannot derive ethical conclusions from meta-physical or theological knowledge of the Good (which we lack) or from a claim that human happiness is the sole good (which we cannot establish)" [30]. His categorical imperative (which he also referred to as the "supreme principle of morality") tested the consistency of maxims or rules by asserting: "I ought never to act except in such a way that I can also will that my maxim become a universal law." On this account, "One must act to treat every person as an end and never as a means only." For Kant, "practical reasoning must reject any principles that cannot be principles for all concerned, which Kant characterizes as non-universalizable principles" [30]. Contemporary Kantian and deontological ethics have many distinct forms [30, 31].

By way of contrast, utilitarian theories strive to maximize beneficial consequences [28, 32]. The principle of utility requires aggregate or collective benefits to be maximized. From an act or rule utilitarian perspective, the principle of utility is the ultimate ethical principle from which all other principles are derived [28]. The utilitarian philosophy developed by Jeremy Bentham (1748–1832) argued that the rightness of an act or policy was determined by the extent to which it would result in the greatest happiness of the greatest number (happiness in the sense of pleasure or absence of pain). This greatest happiness principle has become known as the principle of utility. Bentham's ideas influenced his student John Stuart Mill, who, in his well-known book *On Liberty*, noted that people are more likely to adopt correct beliefs if they are engaged in an open exchange of ideas and encouraged to reexamine and reaffirm their beliefs [33]. Utilitarian philosophies like Mill's are rooted in the notion that an action or policy is right if it leads to the greatest possible balance of good consequences. The goal of finding the greatest good by balancing the interests of all affected persons depends on judgments about likely outcomes [11]. Some utilitarian theories limit the relevant benefits and harms to those experienced by human beings and others include animal species or any entity that can experience benefits and harms [12].

Philosophic moral theories do not arise in a vacuum but rather against a broad background of moral convictions and considered judgments (moral convictions in which we have the highest confidence) [25]. Accounting for a wide range of moral facts provides support for moral theories, which are subject to revisions and improvements [34]. Moral philosophers have expressed skepticism that there will ever be a single philosophic moral theory (e.g., a perfected deductivist theory), that will provide answers to what should be done in all concrete cases [25].

Nondeductivist Principle-Based Approaches

One principle-based approach to moral reasoning has already been mentioned—W. D. Ross's theory of *prima facie* duties [27]. Ross's approach, which emphasizes *prima facie* obligations rather than absolute moral principles or rules, has influenced more recent principle-based approaches that are based on the common morality. Common morality approaches to moral reasoning rely on ordinary shared moral beliefs rather than deduction or pure reason, and may include two or more *prima facie* principles. For example, a common morality theory proposed by William Frankena [35] incorporated principles of beneficence and justice, which are discussed below. The principles of the common morality are viewed as universal standards (analogous to universal human rights) rather than simply local customs, beliefs, and attitudes [11].

The principle-based common morality theory proposed by Beauchamp and Childress [11] was developed to address ethical issues in biomedicine and has not been presented as a comprehensive moral theory. It seeks to reduce morality to its basic elements and to provide a useful framework for ethical analysis in the health professions. The source of the principles is the common morality (socially approved norms of human conduct) and professional norms and traditions in medicine. In Beauchamp and Childress' account, which has frequently been used to analyze ethical issues in public health, principles are abstract and provide only general guides to action. Beneficence, nonmaleficence, respect for autonomy, and justice are included. Only a loose distinction is drawn between rules and principles. What is termed a "coherentist approach" is used for justification of moral judgments and ethical decisions [11]. Simply put, this refers to the coherence of moral arguments and ethical decisions with other rules, principles, and theories.

The ethical principle of *beneficence* requires that potential benefits to individuals and to society be maximized and that potential harms be minimized [11, 28]. Hume referred to benevolence as the "ultimate foundation of morals." In everyday language, beneficence is associated with acts of mercy, charity, and love benefiting other persons [11]. Some beneficent actions are morally required and "others morally discretionary" [36]. The principle of beneficence entails a moral obligation to help other persons (e.g., obligations of health professionals to assist patients) or to provide benefits to others [11]. Beneficence involves both the protection of individual welfare and the promotion of the common welfare.

The principle of *nonmaleficence* requires that harmful acts be avoided. This principle (together with basic rules embedded in the common morality) recognizes that intentionally or negligently causing harm is a fundamental moral wrong [11]. However, the principle of nonmaleficence does not preclude balancing potential harms against potential benefits. For example, the risks and potential harms of medical and public health interventions often must be weighed against possible benefits for patients, research participants, and the public [28].

The principle of *respect for autonomy* focuses on the right of self-determination. This conception of autonomy is not the same as Kant's notion of free will. Autonomy entails freedom from external constraint and the presence of mental capacities needed for understanding and voluntary decision-making [11]. Respect for the autonomy of persons is a principle rooted in the Western tradition, which grants importance to individual freedom in political life, and to personal development [28].

Principles of *justice* are also important [28, 37, 38]. Utilitarian theories of justice emphasize a mixture of criteria so that public utility is maximized. From this perspective, a just distribution of benefits from public programs is determined by the utility to all affected. An egalitarian theory of justice holds that each person should share equally in the distribution of the potential benefits of public services. Other theories of justice hold that society has an obligation to correct inequalities in the distribution of resources, and that those who are least well off should benefit most from available resources. The theory of justice proposed by John Rawls [39] is a leading example of "justice as fairness." Rawls argued that the goal of a theory of justice is to establish the terms of fair cooperation that should govern free and equal moral agents. In this conception, "the appropriate perspective from which to choose among competing conceptions or principles of justice is a hypothetical social contract or choice situation in which contractors are constrained in their knowledge, motivations, and tasks in specific ways." Under constraints of this nature, "rational contractors would choose principles guaranteeing equal basic liberties and equality of opportunity, and a principle that permitted inequalities only if they made the people who are worst off as well off as possible" [40]. Such theories of justice provide considerable support for maximizing benefits to underserved people [37].

The four principles of beneficence, nonmaleficence, justice, and respect for autonomy do not provide an exhaustive account of how the principles can be used as a framework for moral reasoning in biomedicine or public health [11]. The principles also do not provide a full philosophical justification for decision-making. In situations where there is conflict between principles, it may be necessary to choose between them, to assign greater weight to a particular principle, or to further specify principles and rules. Veatch [12] noted that further specification is only one of several approaches that can be considered for resolving conflicts among principles. Other approaches for resolving conflicts include the use of single principle theories (e.g., utilitarianism), balancing theories, conflicting appeals theories, and lexical ordering of principles [12]. Historically, the balancing of principles has been tied to intuition (or, more precisely, what some philosophers refer to as "intuitionism"). The use of balancing theories and intuition to resolve conflicts between principles has the potential drawback of being an elaborate way to provide support for preconceived opinions or prejudices [12]. In the "four-principles" approach to moral reasoning in biomedicine [11], no lexical ordering or ranking of the principles has been proposed.

Ethical decision-making in public health and biomedicine (e.g., decisions about how best to protect participants in human subjects research) require more than merely invoking ethical principles and rules [11]. Through a process of further specification of principles and rules (or another valid approach to resolving conflicts among principles), problems of feasibility, effectiveness, efficiency, uncertainty about benefits and risk, cultural pluralism, political procedures, etc., must also be taken into account [11]. Beauchamp [28] noted that practical problems in biomedical ethics and public policy often require that these principles be made more applicable through a process of specification and reform. Ongoing progressive specification is needed as new issues and concerns arise [41]. The principle-based common morality theory developed by Beauchamp and Childress [11] does not rely on deduction, but rather recognizes that other approaches for justification have value. In various editions of their book, they recognize that moral justification often proceeds inductively (from the particulars of individual cases to more general rules and midlevel principles). Thus, the form of justification they recommend is a coherence approach that is similar to the *reflective equilibrium* described by John Rawls and other philosophers [39, 40, 42]. The connection of the principle-based common morality developed by Beauchamp and Childress to reflective equilibrium appropriately recognizes the dialectical nature of moral reasoning. Seen from this perspective, justification is neither purely *deductivist* nor purely *inductivist*. In Rawls's [39] account, an important starting point is our "considered judgments" or moral convictions in which we have the highest confidence. Considered judgments (sometimes referred to as "self-evident norms and plausible intuitions") are those in which our moral capacities are most likely to be displayed without distortion or bias [11]. A goal of reflective equilibrium, then, is to match and adjust considered judgments and other moral judgments so that they are coherent with the premises of ethical theory. Sound judgment is needed for any method of moral reasoning or ethical decision-making.

Advantages and Limitations of Principle-Based Approaches to Moral Reasoning

Principle-based approaches to moral reasoning, including the method proposed by Beauchamp and Childress for bioethical decision-making, have several advantages [43]. These advantages include their endurance, resilience, and output capacity or yield. A useful philosophical theory or method for moral reasoning should endure through competitive encounters with alternative approaches to moral reasoning, have explanatory power, be adaptive to novel situations, and offer practical solutions to new moral problems [11]. As Beauchamp and Childress put it, "A proposed moral theory is unacceptable if its requirements are so demanding that they probably cannot be satisfied or could be satisfied by only a few extraordinary persons or communities" [11]. Principle-based approaches also have the advantage of universalizability, at least within specific fields such as bioethics and public policy. Universalizability is not a moral norm analogous to a substantive principle of justice but rather a formal conclusion [11]. A further advantage of principle-based approaches to moral reasoning is that they can be joined with a coherence model of justification [11]. Notwithstanding these advantages, principle-based methods of moral reasoning also have certain limitations.

Critiques of these methods for moral reasoning generally occur at the level of metaethics, which involves analysis of the methods and concepts of ethics including general moral principles. Critics of principle-based approaches to moral reasoning have argued that such approaches cannot provide genuine action guides and that they do not provide an adequate philosophical theory [44–47]. Midlevel moral principles function quite differently than fundamental principles do in classical utilitarian (the principle of utility) or Kantian (the categorical imperative) theories [43]. As DeGrazia [44] put it, principlism "acknowledges the lack of a supreme moral principle or set of explicitly-related principles from which all correct moral judgments can be *derived*." Clouser and Gert [46] argued that, in contrast to principle-based approaches in biomedical ethics, principles in deductivist theories such as utilitarianism or Kantian theory summarize or serve as short-hand for a whole theory rather than representing a listing of ethical issues. From this perspective, the four principles of beneficence, autonomy, justice, and nonmaleficence are not systematically related to each other by an underlying unified philosophical theory and there is no priority ranking of the principles [46]. This raises the question of where the principles come from in the first place (a question answered by Beauchamp and Childress by pointing to the common morality and to professional norms and traditions in medicine).

The approach that has been referred to as "principlism," where the emphasis is on general moral principles, has also been criticized for an avoidance of deep engagement with basic theoretical issues in moral theory. In the view of some critics, principle-based approaches are insufficiently attentive to the dialectical relations between philosophical theory and moral practice [45], although others have defended principlism from this criticism [11, 43].

Critics have also charged that the four principles approach to moral reasoning in bioethics, as a version of moral pluralism, suffers from theoretical agnosticism. As Clouser [47] put it, "the principles of principlism are unconnected with each other, and although each embodies the key concern from one or another theory of morality, there is no account of how they should relate to each other." Other authors [11, 43], however, do not agree with this criticism. Beauchamp and Childress [11] noted that there may be a convergence across theories in terms of different theories leading to similar action-guides. Consistent with this viewpoint, DeGrazia [44] argued that the authors of *Principles of Biomedical Ethics* plausibly maintain that two distinct theories (rule-utilitarianism and rule-deontology) are equally adequate. He added, "This pluralistic claim suggests that neither theory itself plays an essential role . . . . We should simply drop these theories from the picture. *The entire network of principles and their specifications becomes the theory*" [44]. Other authors have expressed different perspectives. For example, Brody [48] argued that "We need to understand the theoretical roots of various proposed mid-level principles of bioethics. We need to understand how the theoretical roots do or do not help us to find the scope, implications, and relative significance of the mid-level principles".

A further issue is that some authors have argued that midlevel moral principles may be variously construed, such as when more than one theory of justice is accepted [11]. As DeGrazia [44] put it, "the precise content of the principles is not as crucial as it would be in a deductivist theory. This is because the principles are only starting points; their precise content is determined by specification" [44].

Despite these defenses of the four principles approach and various proposals for further specification, these issues have led some authors to raise important questions about principle-based approaches to biomedical ethics. Green [49] asked, "is it possible in serious discussion of moral issues to bypass entirely any direct consideration of the nature and process of moral justification, the task to which meta-ethics in its most basic effort is devoted?" He further argued "that moral analysis cannot be confined to a process of identifying and applying moral principles, however sophisticated this process might be, when the essential work of deriving the basis, meaning, and scope of these principles is left undone" [49]. To the extent that existing principles and rules are imperfect, coherence between principles and rules will tend to lead to imperfect ethical decisions (analogous to a "bias towards the null" in analytic observational research).

Clouser and Gert [46] have noted that midlevel moral principles such as nonmaleficence collapse four or five moral rules (do not kill, do not cause pain, do not disable, do not deprive of freedom, and do not deprive of pleasure) into a single principle. The principle of autonomy articulated in early editions of *Principles of Biomedical Ethics* (which is quite different from Kant's notion of autonomy) does not distinguish between respecting autonomy and promoting autonomy. Other principles (e.g., the principle of justice) do not provide a specific action guide but rather serve more as a checklist of moral concerns [46]. As Clouser [47] put it, moral conclusions or solutions often seem to be "underdetermined" by the "agent's cited principle." In his view, "There must be other factors (intuitions, rules, theories, or whatever) that are surreptitiously and otherwise influencing the agent's decision-making" [47].

Others have argued that inductive approaches to moral reasoning such as casuistry and analogical reasoning involving particular cases have advantages over principle-based methods [50–53]. From the perspective of casuists such as Albert Jonsen and Stephen Toulmin, neither principle-based methods (which often use a reflective equilibrium or coherence approach for justification) nor philosophic theories based on deductivism adequately express the nature of moral reasoning [50]. Casuists insist that the relation between principles and moral judgment cannot be properly understood without an appreciation of the place of circumstances as integral parts of moral argument [51]. Case materials, casuistry, and analogical reasoning have considerable value for understanding ethics in such diverse fields as medicine, public health, genetics, and the humanities [5, 51–54]. Notwithstanding such potential benefits of case analysis, analogical reasoning does have some disadvantages. For example, casuistry may rely too heavily on intuition in cases of moral conflict [44]. In addition, by focusing on specific cases, casuistry may overlook global ethical issues [44]. Thus, case-based methods of analogical reasoning such as casuistry, as potential alternatives to principle-based methods of moral reasoning, also have certain drawbacks. In addition, principles such as beneficence and respect for autonomy are never far from the maxims (normative statements that reflect a consensus of opinion) and enthymemes that are often invoked in casuistry [51]. Casuistry can be seen as complimentary to principle-based approaches in that the circumstances of cases may suggest the relevance of principles. Also, the circumstances may reveal the suitability of a particular specification of a principle [51].

It is important to note that some earlier criticisms of principle-based methods for moral reasoning have been addressed in revised accounts of these methods. In highlighting inadequacies in principle-based methods for moral reasoning, for example, David DeGrazia [44] asked how one is to know which midlevel principle of biomedical ethics to favor when two or more of autonomy, beneficence, nonmaleficence, and justice conflict? This concern has subsequently been addressed by Beauchamp and Childress in more recent editions of *Principles of Biomedical Ethics* (e.g., in their elaborations of how principles are further specified and moral judgments justified through a coherence approach). Metaethics is dealt with to a greater extent in recent editions of their book. They and other authors have provided accounts of how mid-level moral principles can be further specified in specific contexts [11, 41, 44]. Although different sets of midlevel ethical principles have been proposed by various authors, and definitions of *prima facie* principles vary, this is not problematic if principles are only viewed as starting points for application to specific contexts through further specification [44]. A dialectical relationship exists between fundamental philosophical theories and midlevel principles and rules. On this account, philosophical theory and the application of particular principles and rules in specific contexts serve to enrich and modify one another. As Lustig [43] put it, "theoretical commitments that lead to counterintuitive or implausible conclusions in particular cases may, over time, cast doubt upon the adequacy of one's working theory" and lead to revisions or reassessments of a philosophical theory or method of moral reasoning.

Additional Principles in Public Health Ethics

As noted by Childress et al. [16], "The terrain of public health ethics includes a loose set of general moral considerations—clusters of moral concepts and norms that are variously called values, principles, or rules—that are arguably relevant to public health." Accounts of public health ethics have extended beyond the four commonly cited principles of beneficence, nonmaleficence, respect for the autonomy of persons, and justice to include important rules and values such as ensuring public participation and the participation of affected parties (procedural justice), protecting privacy and confidentiality, keeping promises and commitments, disclosing information and speaking honestly and truthfully (transparency), and building and maintaining public trust [16, 17]. Other rules or conditions cited in the literature on public health ethics include the need for effectiveness, efficiency, proportionality, necessity, least infringement, and public justification [16]. The effectiveness and efficiency of public health programs are closely related to principles of utility and beneficence. The condition or value of transparency, which asserts that government agencies and institutions should be open and transparent in their interactions with the public, is closely tied to moral concepts of veracity and truth telling.

Other examples of principles cited in the public health literature are provided below including the precautionary principle and principles of solidarity or social cohesion. The overall goal of this section is not to detail the complex ethical issues that arise in public health but rather to provide a framework for identifying and clarifying additional principles related to public health ethics, namely, a framework that takes into consideration the interplay of ethical principles and rules at individual, community, national, and global levels.

The Precautionary Principle

In recent decades, there has been sustained interest among environmental ethicists, scientists, and policymakers in the sustainability of the global environment and human systems [55–59]. Sustainability relates to the continuity of the nonhuman environment and to the continuity of social, institutional, and economic aspects of human societies. Biological entities and the nonbiological world (e.g., the atmosphere, land, and ocean) involve complex systems and are fundamentally interdependent. Achieving a sustainable environment is therefore essential to human beings, including future generations. The Brundtland Commission, headed by former Norwegian Prime Minister Gro Harlem Brundtland, defined sustainable development as development that meets the needs of the present without compromising the ability of future generations to meet their own needs. Intergenerational equity underlies concerns over the need to look out for the interests of future generations. This includes taking steps to help ensure that the world inherited by future generations is not diminished by loss of animals, plants, ecosystems, or land that is suitable for homes or growing crops [60].

Concern over the continuity of the global environment and human systems encompasses concern over the sustainability of life and whole ecosystems; economic resources; agricultural and food resources; energy resources; and other natural resources including timber, arable land, and metals or metallic ore. To this list can be added concern over the maintenance or improvement of population health and quality of life. From an analytic standpoint, all of these issues can be examined at the global level and also at smaller levels of analysis (e.g., within geographic regions, countries, states or provinces, cities, or neighborhoods). For example, the sustainability of life and whole ecosystems is a global issue that can also be analyzed from the standpoint of specific geographic regions, countries, and smaller governmental jurisdictions.

From this overview, it is clear that sustainability has multiple dimensions that may be of analytic interest (e.g., focusing on the present and on the future, having a global or more localized frame of reference), and that the concept can be applied to multiple areas of concern that may be interrelated or even conflicting (e.g., concerns over the sustainability of ecosystems sometimes conflict with concerns about economic development). Other dimensions that may be pertinent include the complexity of the human or nonhuman systems of analytic interest, and the degree or extent of sustainability that is desired. Ethical issues that have bearing on the continued functioning of societies (e.g., certain issues that arise in preparedness for natural or man-made disasters) have often been given considerable weight.

The literature on sustainability has led to several questions. For example, what other ethical principles, obligations, and rules relate to it? Some duties are desirable but not obligatory, and others are both morally desirable and obligatory [61]. Rules associated with morally desirable duties, which can be related both to sustainability and to the principle of beneficence, include maximizing possible benefits and balancing benefits against risks. An example of a rule that is both morally desirable and obligatory, which can be related to sustainability and justice, is the requirement that we treat others (including members of future generations) fairly. Rules that can be related to sustainability and non-maleficence include minimizing possible harms and not causing suffering or loss of life. A conceptual understanding of sustainability is useful to public health ethics, especially if it can be shown to provide worthwhile guidance and information above and beyond principles of beneficence, nonmaleficence, and justice, as well as the clusters of existing rules and maxims that are linked to these principles.

The *precautionary principle* asserts that "when an activity raises threats of harm to human health or the environment, precautionary measures should be taken even if some cause and effect relationships are not fully established scientifically." The force of this principle, which relates to the frequent need to take preventive action in the face of scientific uncertainty, is to shift the burden of proof to the proponents of activities that may threaten health or harm the environment [13, 15, 18]. Nevertheless, this principle is not universally accepted by regulatory agencies and policymakers. Critics have argued that it focuses on hypothetical risks rather than actual hazards and that other analytic methods (e.g., cost-benefit analysis) may provide a more suitable basis for regulation. The phrase "precautionary principle" (frequently cited in the literature on environmental advocacy and public policy) is a translation of the German word *Vorsorgeprinzip*, which can also be translated as "foresight principle." The *Vorsorgeprinzip* is often viewed positively among German environmental policymakers as a stimulus for innovative social planning and sustainability [15]. Arguments have been made that *Vorsorgeprinzip* is not a midlevel moral principle, but rather a cluster of virtues (e.g., prudence and wisdom), maxims, and moral rules that can be specified using principles of nonmaleficence, beneficence, and autonomy as starting places (e.g., the rule that a wide range of alternatives to potentially harmful activities should be explored before taking action, and that public participation in decision-making is desirable) [61]. Whether the *Vorsorgeprinzip* is viewed as a "principle" or as a cluster of virtues, maxims, rules, and mid-level moral principles obtained from the common morality, some advocates for public health and the environment may prefer to use the term principle because it gives the concept more thrust or weight.

Connectedness, Solidarity, and Communal Responsibility

The principle of *solidarity* or *social cohesion* provides another useful example of the value of analysis at multiple levels (individual, community, national, and global). This principle relates to how united, connected, and cooperative a society is. A socially cohesive society is one that tolerates and embraces cultural diversity, a society where the vast majority of citizens respect the law and human rights, and where there is a shared commitment to social order and communal responsibility [14, 62]. Many philosophical theories and traditions have attempted to describe the ways in which people are interdependent within communities. *Communitarianism* approaches, for example, draw upon the work of Aristotle and more recent political philosophers (e.g., the writings of Georg Wilhelm Friedrich Hegel) to highlight the importance of tradition and social context for moral reasoning and the value of community. Community can be understood both as a description of human social situations (e.g., the notion of togetherness and solidarity) and as a normative standard for evaluating human situations (e.g., a strong sense of mutual obligation and reciprocity) [14]. Contemporary communitarianism developed in the 1980s in response to concerns about a perceived overemphasis on individual rights. From a communitarian perspective, individuals are inseparable from community life and, although individuals make their own moral choices, their moral commitments and values are shaped by community norms and experiences. As Jennings [14] put it, there is "a fascinating dynamic in which participants are both shaped as selves by their life in community with others and at the same time have the power to reshape their community through their own agency." Communitarians such as Alasdair MacIntyre and Charles Taylor have argued that moral and political judgments such as standards of justice depend on the life contexts and traditions of particular societies and the interpretive framework within which community members view their world [63]. From a communitarian viewpoint, standards of justice and other moral and political judgments may vary from one context to another and not be universally true. Communitarian writers such as Michael Sandel and Charles Taylor have argued that liberal theories of justice such as the one proposed by John Rawls may rest on an overly individualistic conception of the self that does not adequately recognize communal attachments such as family ties, social and communal responsibilities, or religious traditions [63]. Rawls defined community narrowly as "an association of society whose unity rests on a comprehensive conception of the good" [64]. To a greater or lesser extent, communitarian values and principles may conflict with individual autonomy and self-determination [14]. A tension may exist between the liberal tradition that emphasizes individualism and principles of solidarity and social cohesion.

Scientific studies documenting the important role of social support, social networks, and social cohesion in enhancing overall health, well-being, and quality of life provide empirical evidence of the value of social cohesion. For example, studies have shown an association between social connectedness and quality of life and physical functioning among children and adults with a variety of serious illnesses, injuries, and psychological traumas [65–67]. There are important connections between social connectedness and social support and the health, well-being, and resiliency of individuals and whole communities [68, 69]. Some communities or networks of persons may be more resilient and capable of responding positively to adverse events than others, due to differences in community resources, infrastructure, or social and cultural factors [61].

As in the first example, we can reasonably conclude that a principle of solidarity or social cohesion is useful if it provides moral guidance above and beyond existing principles derived from the common morality such as beneficence, nonmaleficence, justice, and respect for the autonomy of persons, including the clusters of rules that are linked to these moral principles. Interactions between principles are likely to be important. For example, the principle of solidarity, when combined with the principle of beneficence and rules linked to it, provides considerable support for building cities with green space, sidewalks, park facilities, and other infrastructure that facilitates exercise and recreation. A growing literature highlights the important role of urban design and architecture in promoting a sense of community, socialization, and improved health and quality of life [70, 71]. Because principles and rules may interact with each other and magnify (or diminish) each other's importance, a simple checklist of principles and rules, in such diverse fields as urban design, city planning, public health, and environmental science, may understate the importance of individual principles and rules for moral reasoning.

Summary and Conclusions

This article has considered general moral principles that play a prominent role in certain methods of moral reasoning in public health and biomedicine, as well as the advantages and disadvantages of methods of moral reasoning that rely on such principles. The taxonomy of principles identified in this account includes principles that figure prominently in some deductivist philosophical theories and midlevel principles based on the common morality. None of the principles in this taxonomy have been confirmed as "first principles" or "ultimate principles" that incontrovertibly fix the foundations of moral reasoning, to paraphrase Hume.

Additional principles cited in the literature on public health ethics were also considered. Ethical principles and values underlie the need to take appropriate action even in the face of some scientific uncertainty [13, 56]. Concepts such as the precautionary principle and solidarity are likely to be useful to public health ethics to the extent that they can be shown to provide worthwhile guidance and information above, and beyond principles of beneficence, nonmaleficence, and justice, and the clusters of rules and maxims linked to these moral principles.

Future directions that are likely to be productive include further work on several areas of public health ethics, including public trust, community empowerment, the rights of individuals who are targeted (or not targeted) by public health interventions (who may include citizens in multicultural democratic societies or in other parts of the world), and individual and community resilience and well-being. Other future directions are likely to include further clarification of principles, obligations, and rules in public health disciplines such as environmental science, prevention and control of chronic and infectious diseases, genomics, and global health [72].

To formulate public policies and decide about particular cases, there will be an ongoing need to further specify and balance the principles using sound judgment [1]. Further specification is viewed as the ongoing process of filling in and development of principles and rules, reducing or eliminating their indeterminateness and abstractness, and providing specific action guides. Sound judgment will be needed to accompany any system of ethical principles and rules. As noted by Aristotle, "It is a task less for the clever arguer than for the *anthropos megalopsychos*, the "large-spirited human being" [73].

Acknowledgment

The findings and conclusions in this article are those of the author and do not necessarily reflect the official position of the Centers for Disease Control and Prevention.

References

1. Beauchamp, T.L. Principlism and Its Alleged Competitors. *Kennedy Inst Ethics J* (1995):5:181–198.
2. Veatch, R.M. How Many Principles for Bioethics? In: Ashcroft, R.E., A. Dawson, H. Draper, and J.R. McMillan, editors, *Principles of Health Care Ethics* (2nd ed.). New York, NY: Wiley (2007):43–50.
3. Beauchamp, T.L., and J.F. Childress. *Principles of Biomedical Ethics* (6th ed.). New York, NY: Oxford University Press (2008).
4. Coughlin, S.S. *Ethics in Epidemiology and Public Health Practice: Collected Works*. Columbus, GA: Quill Publications (1997).
5. Coughlin, S.S., C.L. Soskolne, and K.W. Goodman. *Case Studies in Public Health Ethics*. Washington, D.C.: American Public Health Association (1997).
6. Coughlin, S.S. Ethics in Epidemiologic Research and Public Health Practice. *Emerg Themes Epidemiol* (2006):3:16. Available at http://ete-online.com/content/3/1/16.

 7. Bayer, R., L.O. Gostin, B. Jennings, and B. Steinbock. *Public Health Ethics. Theory, Policy, and Practice*. New York, NY: Oxford University Press (2007).

 8. Susser, M. Falsification, Verification, and Causal Inference in Epidemiology: Reconsiderations in the Light of Sir Karl Popper's Philosophy. In: Rothman, K.J., editor, *Causal Inference*. Chestnut Hill, MA: Epidemiology Resources (1988):33–57.

 9. Rothman, K.J., and S. Greenland. Causation and Causal Inference in Epidemiology. *Am J Public Health* (2005):95:S144–S155.

10. Weed, D.L. Toward a Philosophy of Epidemiology. In: Coughlin, S.S., T.L. Beauchamp, D.L. Weed, editors, *Ethics and Epidemiology* (2nd ed.). New York, NY: Oxford University Press (2009).

11. Beauchamp, T.L., and J.F. Childress. *Principles of Biomedical Ethics* (4th ed.). New York, NY: Oxford University Press (1994).

12. Veatch, R. Resolving Conflicts among Principles: Ranking, Balancing, and Specifying. *Kennedy Inst Ethics J* (1995):199–218.

13. Kriebel, D., and J. Tickner. Reenergizing Public Health through Precaution. *Am J Public Health* (2001):91:1351–1361.

14. Jennings, B. Community in Public Health Ethics. In: Ashcroft, R.E., A. Dawson, H. Draper, and J.R. McMillan, editors, *Principles of Health Care Ethics* (2nd ed.). New York, NY: Wiley (2007):543–548.

15. Callahan, D., and B. Jennings. Ethics and Public Health: Forging a Strong Relationship. *Am J Public Health* (2002):92:169–176.

16. Childress, J.F., R.R. Faden, R.D. Gaare, et al. Public Health Ethics: Mapping the Terrain. *J Law Med Ethics* (2002):30:170–178.

17. Kass, N.E. An Ethics Framework for Public Health. *Am J Public Health* (2001):91:1776–1782.

18. Bayer, R., and A.L. Fairchild. The Genesis of Public Health Ethics. *Bioethics* (2004):18:473–492.

19. Macklin, R. *Against Relativism. Cultural Diversity and the Search for Ethical Universalism in Medicine*. New York, NY: Oxford University Press (1999).

20. Searle, J. *The Construction of Social Reality*. New York, NY: Free Press (1995).

21. Hacking, I. *The Social Construction of What?* Cambridge, MA: Harvard University Press (1999).

22. Hume, D. *Enquiry Concerning the Principles of Morals*. In: Beauchamp, T.L., editor, New York, NY: Oxford University Press (1998).

23. Hume, D. An Enquiry Concerning Human Understanding. In: Beauchamp, T.L., editor, New York, NY: Oxford University Press (1999).

24. Markie, P. Rationalism vs. Empiricism. In: Zalta, N., editor, *The Stanford Encyclopedia of Philosophy* (2004) Available at http://plato.stanford.edu/entries/rationalism-empiricism.

25. Richardson, H.S. Moral Reasoning. In: Zalta, N., editor, *The Stanford Encyclopedia of Philosophy* (2007) Available at http://plato.stanford.edu/entries/reasoning-moral.

26. Dancy, J. Moral Particularism. In: Zalta N, editor, *The Stanford Encyclopedia of Philosophy* (2005) Available at http://plato.stanford.edu/entries/moral-particularism.

27. Ross, W.D. *The Right and the Good*. Oxford: Claredon Press (1930).

28. Beauchamp, T.L. Moral Foundations. In: Coughlin, S.S., and T.L. Beauchamp, editors, *Ethics and Epidemiology*. New York, NY: Oxford University Press (1996):24–52.

29. Kant, I. *Critique of Pure Reason*. In: Guyer, P., and A.W. Wood, editors, New York, NY: Cambridge University Press (1998).

30. O'Neill, O. Kantian Ethics. In: Ashcroft, R.E., A. Dawson, H. Draper, and J.R McMillan, editors, *Principles of Health Care Ethics* (2nd ed.). New York, NY: Wiley (2007):73–77.

31. McNaughton, D.A., and J.P. Rawling. Deontology. In: Ashcroft, R.E., A. Dawson, H. Draper, and J.R. McMillan, editors, *Principles of Health Care Ethics* (2nd ed.). New York, NY: Wiley (2007):65–71.

32. Mill, J.S. Utilitarianism. In: Robson, J.M., editor, *The Collected Works of John Stuart Mill*, vol. X. Toronto: University of Toronto Press (1963).

33. Mill, J.S. On Liberty. In: Robson, J.M., editor, *The Collected Works of John Stuart Mill*. Toronto: University of Toronto Press (1963).

34. Sidgwick, H. *The Methods of Ethics*. Indianapolis, IN: Hackett Publishing (1981).

35. Frankena, W.K. *Ethics* (2nd ed.). Englewood Cliffs, NJ: Prentice Hall (1973).

36. Cullity, G. Beneficence. In: Ashcroft, R.E., A. Dawson, H. Draper, and J.R. McMillan, editors, *Principles of Health Care Ethics* (2nd ed.). New York, NY: Wiley (2007):19–26.

37. Powers, M., and R. Faden. *Social Justice: The Moral Foundations of Public Health and Health Policy*. New York, NY: Oxford University Press (2006).

38. Gostin, L.O., and M. Powers. What Does Social Justice Require for the Public's Health? Public Health Ethics and Policy Imperatives. *Health Affairs (Millwood)* (2006):25:1053–1060.

39. Rawls, J. *A Theory of Justice*. Cambridge, MA: Harvard University Press (1971).

40. Daniels, N. Reflective Equilibrium. In: Zalta, N., editor, *The Stanford Encyclopedia of Philosophy* (2007) Available at http://plato.stanford.edu/entries/reflective-equilibrium.

41. Richardson, H.S. Specifying Norms as a Way to Resolve Concrete Ethical Problems. *Philos Public Aff* (1990):19:279–310.

42. Daniels, N. Wide Reflective Equilibrium and Theory Acceptance in Ethics. *J Philos* (1979):76: 257.

43. Lustig, B.A. The Method of 'Principlism': A Critique of the Critique. *J Med Philos* (1992):17:487–510.

44. DeGrazia, D. Moving Forward in Bioethical Theory: Theories, Cases, and Specified Principlism. *J Med Philos* (1992):17:511–539.

45. Clouser, K.D., and B. Gert. A Critique of Principlism. *J Med Philos* (1990):15:219–236.

46. Clouser, K.D., and B. Gert. Morality vs. Principlism. In: Gillon, R., editor, *Principles of Health Care Ethics*. New York, NY: Wiley (1994).

47. Clouser, K.D. Common Morality as an Alternative to Principlism. *Kennedy Inst Ethics J* (1995):5:219–236.

48. Brody, B.A. Quality of Scholarship in Bioethics. *J Med Philos* (1990):15:161–178.

49. Green, R.M. Method in Bioethics: A Troubled Assessment. *J Med Philos* (1990):15:179–197.

50. Jonsen, A.R., and S.E. Toulmin. *The Abuse of Casuistry*. Berkeley, CA: University of California Press (1988).

51. Jonsen, A.R. Casuistry as Methodology in Clinical Ethics. *Theor Med* (1991):12:299–302.

52. Arras, J.D. Getting Down to Cases: the Revival of Casuistry in Bioethics. *J Med Philos* (1991):16:29–51.

53. Arras, J.D. Principles and Particularity: The Role of Cases in Bioethics. *Indiana Law J* (1994):69:983–1014.

54. Penslar, R.L. *Research Ethics. Cases and Materials*. Indianapolis, IN: Indiana University Press (1995).

55. Brown, D. The Ethical Dimensions of Global Environmental Issues. *Daedalus* (2001):4:59–77.

56. Raffensperger, C., and J. Tickner. *Protecting Public Health and the Environment: Implementing the Precautionary Principle*. Washington, D.C.: Island Press (1999).

57. Attfield, R. *Environmental Ethics: an Overview for the Twenty-First Century*. Cambridge, MA: Polity (2003).

58. Soskolne, C.L., editor. *Sustaining Life on Earth: Environmental and Human Health Through Global Governance*. Lanham, MD: Lexington Books (2007).

59. Coughlin, S.S., C. Bonds, J. Malilay, and J. Araujo. Ethics. In: Golson, J.G., and S.G. Philander, editors, *Encyclopedia of Global Warming and Climate Change*. Thousand Oaks, CA: Sage Publications (2008).

60. Coughlin, S.S. Educational Intervention Approaches to Ameliorate Adverse Public Health and Environmental Effects from Global Warming. *Ethics Sci Environ Polit* (2006):13–14. Available at http://www.int-res.com/articles/esep/2006/E69.pdf.

61. Coughlin, S.S. *The Nature of Principles.* Philadelphia, PA: Xlibris (2008).

62. Heitman, E., and L.C. McKieran. Community-Based Practice and Research: Collaboration and Sharing Power. In: Jennings, B., J. Kahn, A. Mastroianni, and S.L. Parker, editors, *Ethics and Public Health: Model Curriculum.* Washington, D.C.: Association of Schools of Public Health (2003).

63. Taylor, C. *Sources of the Self: The Making of the Modern Identity.* New York, NY: Cambridge University Press (1999).

64. Rawls, J. *Political Liberalism.* New York, NY: Columbia University Press (1993).

65. Dunkel-Schetter, C., L.G. Feinstein, S.E. Taylor, and R.L. Falke. Patterns of Coping with Cancer. *Health Psychol* (1992):11:79–87.

66. Folkman, S., and J. Telie Moskowitz. Coping: Pitfalls and Promise. *Annu Rev Psychol* (2004):55:745–774.

67. Michael, Y.L., L.F. Berkman, G.A. Colditz, et al. Social Networks and Health-Related Quality of Life in Breast Cancer Survivors: A Prospective Study. *J Psychosom Res* (2002):52:285–293.

68. Hardy, S.E., J. Concato, and T.M. Gill. Resilience of Community-Dwelling Older Persons. *J Am Geriatr Soc* (2004):52:257–262.

69. Jackson, J.M., S.J. Rolnick, S.S. Coughlin, et al. Social Support among Women Who Died of Ovarian Cancer. *Support Care Cancer* (2007):15:547–556.

70. Hall, P. *Cities of Tomorrow: An Intellectual History of Urban Planning and Design in the Twentieth Century* (3rd ed.). Oxford: Blackwell (2002).

71. Partners for Livable Cities. *The Livable City: Revitalizing Urban Communities.* New York, NY: McGraw-Hill (2000).

72. Coughlin, S.S. Ethical Issues in Epidemiology. In: Ashcroft, R., A. Dawson, H. Draper, and J. McMillian, editors, *Principles of Health Care Ethics.* London: Wiley (2007):601–606.

73. Wheelwright, P., translator. *Aristotle: The Nicomachean Ethics.* New York, NY: Odyssey Press (1951).

PART III

THE ETHICS OF EPIDEMIOLOGIC RESEARCH AND PUBLIC HEALTH PRACTICE

The societal importance of public health activities including epidemiology has contributed to current interest in ethical issues in public health practice and research including issues well known to many practicing epidemiologists. Public health measures include the collection and analysis of epidemiologic data, evaluative research, and health promotion and disease prevention activities. The determinants of population health are multifactorial (e.g., biological, behavioral, social, and environmental) in that such factors may influence health and interact at multiple levels (e.g., at the level of individuals, communities, or societies).

Ethical concerns in epidemiology and public health practice often relate to the obligations of health professionals to acquire and apply scientific knowledge aimed at maintaining and restoring public health while respecting individual rights. Potential societal benefits must often be balanced with risks and potential harms to individuals and communities such as invasions of privacy or the potential for stigmatization. Many public health measures (e.g., requirements that physicians report cases of certain communicable diseases and provisions for vaccinating children against infectious diseases) are legally mandated. Public health practitioners must often balance the need to promote the common welfare against individual rights to autonomy or expectations of privacy.

The articles included in this section of the book highlight ethical and professional norms in epidemiology as well as ethical issues arising in public health practice. As the following articles explain, important distinctions must be drawn between epidemiologic research and areas of public health practice such as surveillance systems, outbreak investigations, emergency preparedness and response, and evaluation studies in identifying ethical responsibilities. Ethical issues in one area of public health practice—disease surveillance—are illustrated using examples from the field of cancer registration.

Some of the issues discussed in this section are "bread and butter" ethical issues arising in research with human research participants (e.g., those pertaining to informed consent) and issues well known to public health practitioners (e.g., the need to rigorously safeguard the confidentiality of information included in surveillance systems). Other issues discussed in this section, such as those at the intersection of organizational ethics and public health practice, are just beginning to be discussed in the published literature.

CHAPTER 4

ETHICALLY OPTIMIZED STUDY DESIGNS IN EPIDEMIOLOGY

Steven S. Coughlin

It is generally accepted that epidemiologists have a moral and professional obligation to maximize the potential benefits of research studies to subjects and to society, and to minimize potential risks, as enjoined by the ethical principle of beneficence (which requires providing benefits and balancing benefits against risks) [1, 2]. An example is found in the rule that the confidentiality of medical information used in epidemiologic research should be conscientiously protected [3–5]. Other moral obligations of epidemiologists are grounded in the principle of nonmaleficence (which requires that we avoid causing harm), a principle that has often been associated with the Hippocratic injunction to do no harm [1, 2]. For example, in carrying out studies in developing countries, there is a need to avoid harming members of impoverished communities by diverting scarce health personnel from their routine activities in order to meet the needs of research studies [6].

Epidemiologists also have an obligation to respect the autonomy of individuals who participate in research studies, a principle that underlies rules of privacy and confidentiality. These rules should not be violated without first obtaining the informed consent of research subjects, except under exceptional circumstances when that is impractical and the potential risks and benefits of the research have been carefully considered by an independent review committee [1, 5]. A further obligation is the need to ensure that the burdens and benefits of epidemiologic research are distributed in an equitable fashion, which is grounded in ethical principles of justice (principles of fairness in the distribution of benefits and risks) [2]. Recent efforts to ensure that women and minorities are adequately represented in research projects funded by the National Institutes of Health (NIH) are well-known examples [7].

As these illustrations suggest, the ethical principles of beneficence, nonmaleficence, justice, and respect for autonomy provide a useful framework through which many moral problems surrounding epidemiology may be understood and evaluated. Careful specification of these principles helps ensure that the welfare and rights of individuals and communities are protected in the design and conduct of epidemiologic studies [2, 8]. Furthermore, these principles are reflected in ethics guidelines for epidemiologists such as those developed by the Council of International Organizations of Medical Sciences, the International Epidemiological Association, and the Industrial Epidemiology Forum [9–11]. Specific understandings of these principles have contributed to the presentation below, although this chapter does not overtly reflect or engage in the type of philosophical argument that analyzes or specifies these principles.

"Ethically Optimized Study Designs in Epidemiology" originally appeared in Ethics and Epidemiology. New York: Oxford University Press (1996). Used with permission of Oxford University Press, Inc.

With the possible exception of safeguards for protecting privacy and the confidentiality of information obtained from research subjects, there has been inadequate discussion of specific recommendations that can be made to ensure that epidemiologic studies are ethically optimized. In the discussion that follows, specific improvements in design are considered that may minimize potential risks to subjects and groups of individuals, maximize the potential benefits of nonexperimental epidemiologic studies to individuals and to communities, and increase the likelihood that the benefits and burdens of the research are distributed in an equitable fashion. The adequacy of provisions for obtaining the informed consent of subjects is also considered below in relation to epidemiologic study design.

Minimizing Risks to Subjects and Groups

The risks posed by nonexperimental epidemiologic studies are often minor compared with those that must be considered in designing and conducting clinical trials and other experimental studies, and surveys of respondents' attitudes toward participation in epidemiologic studies have suggested that many subjects find the experience personally satisfying or rewarding [12, 13]. Nevertheless, individuals participating in epidemiologic research may be burdened by a loss of privacy (the condition of limited access to a person), by time spent completing interviews and undergoing examinations, and, in some instances, by adverse psychological effects such as anxiety and grief [2]. Other potential risks in some studies include stigmatization and loss of employment or insurance resulting from breaches of confidentiality, although these are admittedly remote possibilities in most epidemiologic studies because of regulatory controls and organizational safeguards [14]. On the other hand, there may be risks to privacy from disclosure of confidential information to third parties in the institution at which the research is conducted.

Measures that may be taken to protect individual privacy and ensure the confidentiality of health information are well known to most epidemiologists. Examples of such protective measures include keeping records with personal identifiers under lock and key, limiting access to confidential records to selected members of the research team on a need-to-know basis, discarding personal identifiers from data collection forms and computer files whenever feasible, reinforcing the importance of maintaining the confidentiality of health records at the time of orientation and training sessions for study personnel, and various safeguards to prevent data from publication or release in a form that would allow previously undisclosed identifications to occur [3, 4, 15].

In addition to measures for ensuring confidentiality, a number of other specific steps may be taken to minimize risks to individuals participating in epidemiologic studies. For example, potential risks and inconveniences may be reduced by restricting the length of questionnaires and examinations, by allowing maximum flexibility in scheduling interviews, and by not scheduling interviews on holidays or anniversary dates that are likely to enhance grief [2]. It may also be important to postpone surrogate interviews until after a reasonable amount of time has elapsed since the death of the respective family member.

Although such protective measures may currently be widely practiced in epidemiology, exceptions do occur. For example, in a case-control study of sudden infant death syndrome in two counties in Great Britain, the parents of deceased infants were interviewed within 72 hours of their child's death, most within 24 hours [16]. The parents were questioned about social factors, family history, maternal medical history, details of the pregnancy and perinatal period, and the infant's medical history, including recent signs of illness, feeding habits, precise details of the infant's last sleep, the position in which he or she had been found, the precise quantity and nature of the clothing and bedding, whether the baby had been swaddled, whether the bedclothes had been over the baby's head when found, how the baby's room was heated, and the time the heat had been on [16].

It might be argued that any psychological distress resulting from participation in studies of this nature is likely to be relatively minor and transitory, and that the potential social benefits of the study must also be taken into account. Furthermore, the reliability and validity of some information obtained from next-of-kin are likely to decline over time. However, principles such as beneficence and respect for autonomy suggest that recently bereaved individuals and other vulnerable populations are deserving of protective measures such as obtaining epidemiologic data in a less intrusive fashion. The principle of nonmaleficence, which demands the noninfliction of harmful acts that may impair health or lead to mental distress [1, 2], also bears on this discussion, although nonmaleficence—when conjoined with the principle of beneficence—does not preclude balancing potential harms against potential benefits. Other case-control studies of sudden infant death syndrome have examined similar associations while delaying interviews of bereaved parents until 6 weeks after their baby's death [17]. Prospective studies of high-risk infants have also been undertaken [18], and such studies may avoid the need to interview recently bereaved parents.

Furthermore, epidemiologic research can inadvertently pose potential risks to groups of individuals and communities. For example, populations defined by race, ethnicity, or lifestyle may suffer stigmatization or lowered self-image following the publication and dissemination of research findings that create or reinforce negative cultural stereotypes [19, 20]. A related problem is the way in which epidemiologic research findings are presented to the public by the media. For example, shortly after the initial reports of an epidemic of respiratory distress syndrome among adults residing in the American Southwest, the *Washington Post* reported concern among Navajos that inaccurate talk of a "Navajo Flu," or more broadly "Navajo illness," might lead to unfounded efforts to segregate or otherwise avoid contact with that community [21]. Disparaging information about a group can result in harms such as discrimination in employment, housing, or insurance, or lowered self-esteem and racial or cultural pride [19]. The problems encountered by Haitians following their identification as a risk group for human immunodeficiency virus (HIV) infection and AIDS further illustrates such harms [20, 22].

As an example of how risks to groups can be minimized through improvements in study design, epidemiologic studies of racial or ethnic differences in disease associations or risk factors can sometimes adopt more scientifically valid measures of income, educational attainment, and other indices of socioeconomic status. This enables investigators to better examine whether socioeconomic factors or other exposures account for any observed associations with race or ethnicity [23]. In some instances, it may also be desirable to apply statistical methods that correct risk estimates for imprecision in the assessment of exposure variables [24, 25] or to present findings using alternative classifications such as socioeconomic status or geographic locality, particularly when this is both scientifically and ethically defensible [20, 26].

The identification of disparities in health or the maldistribution of health services across groups defined by race, ethnicity, or lifestyle can serve as a basis for health planning and policymaking, and thereby contribute to improving the health of those who are less well-off in society [27]. For example, surveys have suggested that lesbians may be more likely to develop cancer of the breast as a result of reproductive decisions, increased alcohol consumption and body mass, underutilization of screening mammography, and attitudinal, economic, and provider-related barriers to receiving quality preventive health care [28–30]. However, few surveys of lesbian health practices have been undertaken and scientifically valid data with which to plan cancer-control interventions in this possible high-risk population are currently limited. Indeed, data from the Surveillance, Epidemiology, and End Results cancer registries [31] and most large-scale epidemiologic studies of women do not include information about sexual orientation. In view of the overwhelming evidence that sexual orientation and sexual activity are related to health behaviors and risk factors for disease, the absence of questions about sexual orientation in many large-scale epidemiologic studies seems unscientific. Of course, decisions to include questions about sexual orientation must take into account concerns about privacy and the *possible* impact of such questions on response rates.

It is also conceivable that studies of the health practices of lesbians could inadvertently contribute to discrimination against them in employment or insurance. For example, some early surveys of lesbians were limited to small samples of women encountered at bars—an approach likely to introduce study bias and to convey negative impressions of this diverse community of women. Such risks can be minimized by ensuring that scientifically valid sampling procedures are used, similar to those applied in more recent surveys of lesbians and gay men [28, 32]. In some studies, it may also be helpful to include questions about sexual activity rather than orientation, to avoid the need for labeling respondents according to their sexual orientation. For example, in interviews asked as part of the Women's Health Initiative, the respondents were asked if they are sexually active and, if so, whether they prefer having sex with men, women, or both.

As this example illustrates, epidemiologic research does not take place in a social vacuum, and areas of ethical conflict may exist between the need to obtain scientifically accurate information about the health of population subgroups and the moral imperative to avoid harming populations that already suffer stigmatization and discrimination from the mainstream societies in which they live [22]. Many competing values may have moral weight equal to or greater than the freedom of scientific inquiry. Which values should be put in the balance and how much weight they should be given will often be controversial, and a consensus may not emerge. Nonetheless, developments such as the decision by the NIH Office of Women's Health to designate lesbians as a population subgroup worthy of further study, suggest that these challenges can be met and that positive professional and social change is possible.

Maximizing Benefits to Subjects and to Society

The potential benefits of epidemiologic research are largely societal in nature and include obtaining new information about the etiology and preventive aspects of important causes of morbidity and mortality, and about the utilization of health care resources [27, 33]. The promotion of the common good is an important aspect of beneficence and provides strong justification for many public health measures [1, 34]. The individuals who participate in epidemiologic studies often derive no direct benefit from the research [33]. Nevertheless, opportunities sometimes exist for subjects to receive some personal gain from participation, such as when previously unrecognized disease is detected during health examinations and individuals are then referred to private physicians for treatment [27].

Many other opportunities exist to maximize the usefulness of epidemiologic studies. One example concerns a multicenter epidemiologic study of HIV infection in women in the Washington, D.C. area as part of the Women's Interagency Health Study. The investigators agreed to provide previously unavailable data on the health care utilization of these women to the D.C. Commission of Public Health (with personal identifiers removed) in order to assist the D.C. Office of AIDS Activities in planning and allocating future AIDS services to area residents. In view of the cost of many epidemiologic studies and the increasing scarcity of health care resources, such opportunities to extend the potential benefits of epidemiologic research to local communities should not be overlooked.

A further area in which improvements in study design may maximize the potential benefits of epidemiologic research is the combination of large observational studies with randomized clinical trials. For example, in a multicenter study by the Vaginal Infections and Prematurity Study Group, an observational study of *Ureaplasm urealyticum* among 8,287 pregnant women was followed by a randomized controlled trial of erythromycin for the prevention of premature delivery [35]. Women who had *U. urealyticum* discovered at the screening visit and who were eligible for enrollment in the trial were asked to sign a second informed consent form [35]. By combining observational and randomized study designs, the investigators increased the likelihood that some subjects would benefit from the research, and decreased the likelihood that clinical practice would be inappropriately changed due to the dissemination of observational research findings alone. Although the results of the trial were negative, this study still illustrates how the efficiency of epidemiologic research can be enhanced—and potential benefits to subjects and to society maximized—through the use of innovative study designs.

As part of some population-based studies, it may be feasible to plan some health care advantage to the community following completion of the study, such as epidemiologic research that leads to the establishment of a local disease registry or the training of members of a community in basic methods of population research [20]. The indirect benefits of epidemiologic studies may be particularly important to consider in planning and carrying out studies in socioeconomically disadvantaged populations, such as research conducted in some developing countries and in some urban and rural areas of the United States.

A Just Distribution of the Burdens and Benefits of Research

The historical practice of relying on patients treated at inner-city teaching hospitals for experimental studies has been criticized since low-income minority patients tend to be overrepresented and therefore bear a greater share of the potential risks of the research [2]. Such arguments call upon an egalitarian theory of justice, which implies that each person or class of persons in society should receive an equal share of the potential burdens (and benefits) of health research [1, 2]. Different considerations may apply to epidemiologic research because the risks associated with nonexperimental studies are relatively minor, and the evidence suggests that, if anything, minority populations were often underrepresented in epidemiologic studies until recently [2]. Nonetheless, the potential risks and benefits of epidemiologic studies to different social subgroups are partly determined by the nature of the study population and the generalizability of the findings. To cite one example, most studies of factors associated with survival in idiopathic dilated cardiomyopathy have been carried out in predominately Caucasian patient populations, and little is known about racial differences in mortality in idiopathic dilated cardiomyopathy [36]. Results from the Washington, D.C.,

Dilated Cardiomyopathy Study suggest that black patients with this poorly understood cause of heart failure may be substantially more likely to die in the first 2 years following diagnosis than are whites, even after other prognostic factors are taken into account [36].

Studies that draw their subjects from an entire community or geographic locality, such as the Bogalusa Heart Study [37] and the Atherosclerosis Risk in Communities Study [38], are more likely to distribute the benefits and burdens of research equitably than are studies of relatively selected patient populations. Studies selecting subjects from several hospitals in an attempt to reduce referral bias and increase the representativeness of the sample may also treat subjects more equitably [2].

Obtaining Informed Consent

A further consideration in designing epidemiologic studies is the adequacy of provisions for obtaining the informed consent of subjects. The ability of individuals to reach an autonomous decision regarding their participation in a research study may be diminished during hospitalization as a result of illness, medication, or dependence on physicians and other health care providers [1]. For example, patients may feel obligated to participate in the study or feel that their relationship with their physician will be harmed by failure to participate, even when their right to withhold consent is carefully explained to them. Individuals are therefore motivated to do something they wish not to do, even though the agent seeking a consent does not intend to so manipulate them.

In light of this observation, when feasible it is both prudent and respectful to request consent from potential subjects only after they have recovered or have been discharged from the hospital. The informed consent of individuals who have already been discharged from the hospital may be obtained verbally over the telephone, or by mailing a consent form to their home address. The informed consent of nonhospitalized individuals may also be obtained in person if the interviews are conducted in the subjects' homes. A further issue is whether the quality of informed consent obtained by telephone or in person is likely to be increased or diminished. Written informed consent statements are easier for some individuals to understand, but not for others.

A case-control study of breast cancer and exposure to hair dye carried out at the Sloan-Kettering Cancer Center illustrates several issues about informed consent [39]. The subjects were interviewed in the hospital during the course of their admission. Interviews were obtained from 89.5% of 448 eligible cases, and 92.6% of 675 eligible hospital controls who were primarily women with other types of cancer [39]. The most common reasons for refusal given by nonconsenting subjects were "too many interviews," "too ill," and "don't like to be interviewed." The scientific validity of this study was enhanced by showing the subjects photographs of hair dye brands as a memory aid. If the subjects had been interviewed at home following discharge, by telephone or in person, their ability to reach an autonomous decision regarding participation in the study might have been improved, but alternative interviewing procedures of this nature might have been overly costly or logistically difficult, and telephone interviews would not have allowed for the use of visual aids. Nevertheless, in other case-control studies of this association, the subjects have been interviewed at home by telephone. For example, in a study by Nasca et al. [40], telephone interviews were obtained for 96% (118 of 123) of patients with breast cancer. However, the response rate among the potential neighborhood controls identified by random digit dialing was only 77%.

Some patients have such limited knowledge bases that communication about alien or novel situations is difficult, especially if new concepts are involved [41]. But even under difficult circumstances, enhanced understanding and adequate decisions are often possible. Successful communication of unfamiliar and specialized information to laypersons can often be accomplished by drawing analogies between new information and more ordinary events familiar to them [41]. Similarly, professionals can express risks in both numeric and nonnumeric probabilities through comparison with more familiar risks and prior experiences.

At the same time, obligations to obtain informed consent have limits. Consent requirements imposed by institutions should be formulated and evaluated against a range of social and institutional considerations. The preservation of autonomous choice is the first, but certainly not the only, consideration. For example, a patient's need for education and counseling to achieve a substantial understanding of a medical situation must be balanced against the interests of other patients and of society in maintaining a productive and efficient health care system [41]. Accordingly, institutional policies must consider what is fair and reasonable to require of health care professionals and researchers, what the effect would be of alternative consent requirements on efficiency and effectiveness in the advancement of science, and—particularly in medical care—what the effect of the requirements would be on the welfare of patients. Nowhere is this problem better illustrated than in epidemiology.

Summary and Conclusions

This chapter has considered a number of steps that may be taken in the design and conduct of nonexperimental epidemiologic studies to ensure that such studies are ethically optimized. Although some of the suggested improvements in design exceed the minimum regulatory requirements of many institutional review boards and funding agencies, they are still morally defensible and, at the very least, consistent with morally justified procedures in the conduct of epidemiologic science. Of course, some of the recommended study design elements may already be commonly practiced in epidemiology, or may not be practical in all research settings.

This overview has drawn from a rich and growing literature on the ethics of epidemiologic research, including recently formulated ethics guidelines for epidemiologists [9–11]. Nevertheless, existing guidelines do not provide an exhaustive set of specific recommendations for how epidemiologists can best meet their obligations to identify solutions to important public health problems, while protecting their subjects from morally inappropriate requests and methods.

References

1. Beauchamp, T.L., and J.F. Childress. *Principles of Biomedical Ethics* (4th ed.). New York, NY: Oxford University Press (1994).
2. Coughlin, S.S., and T.L. Beauchamp. Ethics, Scientific Validity, and the Design of Epidemiologic Studies. *Epidemiology* (1992):3:343–347.
3. Gordis, L., E. Gold, and R. Seltser. Privacy Protection in Epidemiologic and Medical Research: a Challenge and a Responsibility. *Am J Epidemiol* (1977):105:163–168.
4. Kelsey, J.L. Privacy and Confidentiality in Epidemiological Research Involving Patients. *IRB* (1981):3:1–4.

5. McCarthy, C.R., and J.P. Porter. Confidentiality: the Protection of Personal Data in Epidemiological and Clinical Research Trials. *Law, Medicine and Health Care* (1991):19:238–241.

6. Council for International Organizations of Medical Sciences. International Guidelines for Ethical Review of Epidemiological Studies. *Law, Medicine and Health Care* (1991):19:247–258.

7. U.S. House of Representatives, Committee on Energy and Commerce. National Institutes of Health Revitalization Amendments of 1990 (report 101-869). Washington, D.C.: U.S. Government Printing Office (1990).

8. Weed, D.L., and S.S. Coughlin. Ethics in Cancer Prevention and Control. In: Greenwald, P., B.F. Kramer, and D.L. Weed, editors, *Cancer Prevention and Control*, New York, NY: Marcel-Dekker (1995).

9. Bankowski, Z., J.H. Bryant, and J.M. Last, editors. Ethics and Epidemiology: International Guidelines. *Proceedings of the XXVth Council for International Organizations of Medical Sciences Conference*, November 7–9, 1990 (summary of discussions). Geneva: CIOMS (1991):137–142.

10. American Public Health Association. *Epidemiology Section Newsletter* (winter 1990).

11. Beauchamp, T.L., R.R. Cook, W.E. Fayerweather, et al. Ethical Guidelines for Epidemiologists. *J Clin Epidemiol* (1991):44:151S–169S.

12. Savitz, D.A., R.F. Hamman, C. Grace, et al. Respondents Attitudes Regarding Participation in an Epidemiologic Study. *Am J Epidemiol* (1986):123:362–366.

13. Taylor, C., P. Trowbridge, and C. Chilvers. Stress and Cancer Surveys: Attitudes of Participants in a Case-Control Study. *J Epidemiol Commun Health* (1991):45:317–320.

14. Greenwald, R.A, M.K. Ryan, and J.E. Mulvihill, editors. *Human Subjects Research: A Handbook for Institutional Review Boards*. New York, NY: Plenum Press (1982).

15. NCHS Staff Manual on Confidentiality. Hyattsville, MD: National Center for Health Statistics (1984) DHSS publication no. (PHS) 84-1244.

16. Fleming, P.J., R. Gilbert, Y. Azaz, et al. Interaction between Bedding and Sleeping Position in the Sudden Infant Death Syndrome: A Population Based Case-Control Study. *Br Med J* (1990):301:85–89.

17. Ponsonby, A.L., T. Dwyer, L.E. Gibbons, et al. Thermal Environment and Sudden Infant Death Syndrome: Case-Control Study. *Br Med J* (1992):304:277–282.

18. Gibbons, L.E., A.L. Ponsonby, and T. Dwyer. A Comparison of Prospective and Retrospective Responses on Sudden Infant Death Syndrome by Case and Control Mothers. *Am J Epidemiol* (1993):137:654–659.

19. Gostin, L. Ethical Principles for the Conduct of Human Subject Research: Population-Based Research and Ethics. *Law, Medicine and Health Care* (1991):19:191–201.

20. Dickens, B.M. Issues in Preparing Ethical Guidelines for Epidemiological Studies. *Law, Medicine and Health Care* (1991):19:175–183.

21. "Navajos Fight Fear with Faith. Tribe Shadowed by Strange Illness," *The Washington Post* (June 3, 1993):1.

22. Dickens, B.M., L. Gostin, and R.J. Levine. Research on Human Populations: National and International Ethical Guidelines. *Law, Medicine and Health Care* (1991):19:157–161.

23. Stern, M.P. Invited Commentary: Do Risk Factors Explain Ethnic Differences in Type II Diabetes? *Am J Epidemiol* (1993):137:733–734.

24. Kleinbaum, D.G., L.L. Kupper, and H. Morgenstern. *Epidemiologic Research. Principles and Quantitative Methods*. Belmont, CA: Lifetime Learning Publications (1982) pp. 220–41.

25. Rosner, B., D. Spiegelman, and W.C. Willett. Correction of Logistic Regression Relative Risk Estimates and Confidence Intervals for Measurement Error: the Case of Multiple Covariates Measured with Error. *Am J Epidemiol* (1990):132:734–745.

26. Freeman, H. Race, Poverty, and Cancer (Editorial). *J National Cancer Inst* (1991):83:551–557.

27. Last, J.M. Epidemiology and Ethics. *Law, Medicine and Health Care* (1991):19:166–174.
28. Bradford, J., and C. Ryan. The National Lesbian Health Care Survey. National Gay and Lesbian Health Foundation (1987).
29. Bybee, D. Michigan Lesbian Health Survey. Michigan Organization for Human Rights (1990).
30. Warchafsky, L. Lesbian Health Needs Assessment. Los Angeles Gay and Lesbian Community Services Center (1992).
31. Miller, B.A., L.A.G. Ries, B.F. Hankey, et al. *Cancer Statistics Review, 1973–1989.* Bethesda: National Cancer Institute (1992) NIH publication no. 92-2789.
32. Munoz, A., L.K. Schrager, H. Bacellar, et al. Trends in the Incidence of Outcomes Defining Acquired Immunodeficiency Syndrome (AIDS) in the Multicenter AIDS Cohort Study: 1985–1991. *Am J Epidemiol* (1993):137:423–438.
33. Gordis, L. Ethical and Professional Issues in the Changing Practice of Epidemiology. *J Clin Epidemiol* (1991):44:9S–13S.
34. Lappé, M. Ethics and Public Health. In: Last, J.M., editor, *Public Health and Preventive Medicine* (12th ed.). Norwalk, CT: Appleton-Century-Crofts (1986):1867–1877.
35. Eschenbach, D.A., R.P. Nugent, A.V. Rao, et al. A Randomized Placebo-Controlled Trial of Erythromycin for the Treatment of *Ureaplasma urealyticum* to Prevent Premature Delivery. *Am J Obstet Gynecol* (1991):164:734–742.
36. Coughlin, S.S., J.S. Gottdiener, K.L. Baughman, et al. Black–White Differences in Mortality in Idiopathic Dilated Cardiomyopathy: The Washington, DC Dilated Cardiomyopathy Study. *J Natl Med Assoc* (1994):86:583–591.
37. Berenson, G.S., S.R. Srinivasan, L.S. Webber, et al. Cardiovascular Risk in Early Life: the Bogalusa Heart Study. In: *Current Concepts.* Kalamazoo, MI: The Upjohn Co. (1991).
38. The ARIC investigators. The Atherosclerosis Risk in Communities (ARIC) Study: Design and Objectives. *Am J Epidemiol* (1989):129:687–702.
39. Wynder, E.L., and M. Goodman. Epidemiology of Breast Cancer and Hair Dyes. *J Natl Cancer Inst* (1983):71:481–488.
40. Nasca, P.C., C.E. Lawrence, P. Greenwald, et al. Relationship of Hair Dye Use, Benign Breast Disease, and Breast Cancer. *J Natl Cancer Inst* (1980):64:23–28.
41. Faden, R.R., and T.L. Beauchamp. *A History and Theory of Informed Consent.* New York, NY: Oxford University Press (1986).

CHAPTER 5

ETHICAL ISSUES IN EPIDEMIOLOGIC RESEARCH AND PUBLIC HEALTH PRACTICE

Steven S. Coughlin

A rich and growing body of literature has emerged on ethics in epidemiologic research and public health practice [1–11]. Recent articles have included conceptual frameworks of public health ethics and overviews of historical developments in the field [7, 8, 11]. Several important topics in public health ethics have also been highlighted [7, 11, 12].

This article provides an overview of ethical issues in epidemiologic research and public health practice for readers who do not necessarily have an in-depth knowledge of public health ethics. In the discussion that follows, a summary is provided of current definitions and conceptualizations of public health ethics and key ethical concerns in the field.

Definitions and Conceptualizations of Public Health Ethics

The starting point for conceptualizations of public health ethics has often been general definitions of public health, such as the definition provided by the Institute of Medicine in 1988: "Public health is what we, as a society, do collectively to assure the conditions in which people can be healthy." As noted by Childress et al. [8], "Public health is primarily concerned with the health of the entire population, rather than the health of individuals. Its features include an emphasis on the promotion of health and the prevention of disease and disability; the collection and use of epidemiological data, population surveillance, and other forms of empirical quantitative assessment; a recognition of the multidimensional nature of the determinants of health; and a focus on the complex interactions of many factors—biological, behavioral, social, and environmental—in developing effective interventions." Public health activities also include community collaborations and partnerships for health and the identification of priorities for public health action.

Previous authors have identified ethical issues and core values in public health, and highlighted differences and similarities between public health ethics and other areas of bioethics [5, 7]. Public health ethics, which can be defined as the identification, analysis, and resolution of ethical problems arising in public health practice and research, has

"Ethical Issues in Epidemiologic Research and Public Health Practice" originally appeared in Emerging Themes in Epidemiology (2006):3:16doi:10.1186/1742-7622-3-16. http://www.ete-online.com/content/3/1/16

different domains from those of medical ethics. Ethical concerns in public health often relate to the dual obligations of public health professionals to acquire and apply scientific knowledge aimed at restoring and protecting the public's health while respecting individual autonomy [1, 3]. Ethics in public health involves an interplay between protecting the welfare of the individual, as in medicine, and the public health goal of protecting the public welfare [1]. Other ethical concerns in public health relate to the need to ensure a just distribution of public health resources [13]. Public health ethics has a broad scope that includes ethical and social issues arising in health promotion and disease prevention, epidemiologic research, and public health practice [5, 7].

In conceptualizing public health ethics and distinguishing it from other areas of bioethics, previous authors have often highlighted mandatory or coercive public health measures that are authorized by public health law (e.g., quarantining people with contagious diseases) or activities that may infringe upon personal privacy or autonomy, such as public health surveillance. In many public health activities, there is a tension between concerns over personal liberties and individual autonomy and public health perspectives, which may be utilitarian, paternalistic, or communitarian. Communitarian perspectives may favor limiting individual autonomy for the sake of the common good or public interest [7].

Despite the importance of mandatory public health activities required by law, many examples of voluntary public health activities can be cited. Public health surveys, for instance, depend on the support and informed consent of members of the public. In deliberating about ethical questions in their own public health activities, public health professionals have increasingly referred to explications of moral reasoning methods useful for public health research and practice.

Moral Reasoning in Public Health

Moral reasoning involves deliberating about ethical questions and reaching a decision with the help of judgment and rational analysis. In such deliberations, particular decisions and actions may be justified by ethical theory or an integrated body of rules and principles. Two theories have commonly been cited in public health research and practice: deontological and utilitarian [14]. Deontological theories (sometimes referred to as Kantian theories) hold that people should not be treated as means to an end and that some actions are right or wrong regardless of the consequences. Deontological theories provide strong support for protecting research participants and whole communities of people, even if protections for human subjects slow research or the acquisition of knowledge.

Utilitarian theories, on the other hand, strive to maximize beneficial consequences. The principle of utility requires aggregate or collective benefits to be maximized. From a utilitarian perspective, the principle of utility is the ultimate ethical principle from which all other principles are derived [14]. Utilitarian theories provide strong justification for public health programs such as mandatory vaccination programs for children and the fluoridation of public water supplies.

Different methods of moral reasoning have been applied to ethical decision-making in public health research and practice [5]. Two approaches have figured most prominently: the principle-based approach to moral reasoning explicated by Beauchamp and Childress [17], and case-based methods such as casuistry [15].

Principle-Based Approaches

Principle-based approaches to moral reasoning were developed to address ethical issues in clinical medicine and are not necessarily the optimal approach for analyzing ethical issues in public health. The four principles of beneficence, nonmaleficence, justice, and respect for autonomy are mentioned in ethics guidelines drafted for public health professionals, although the guidelines do not provide an exhaustive account of how the principles can be used as a framework for ethical decision-making [9, 16]. Principles such as justice also figure prominently in still-evolving ethics frameworks that have been proposed for public health [8, 11, 13].

The principles of beneficence, nonmaleficence, autonomy, and justice, as explained by Beauchamp and Childress [17], seek to reduce morality to its basic elements and to provide a useful framework for ethical analysis in the health professions. The principles do not provide a full philosophical justification for decision-making, however. In situations where there is conflict between principles, it may be necessary to choose between them or to assign greater weight to one. Practical problems in public health ethics require that these principles be made more applicable through a process of specification and reform [14]. Ongoing progressive specification is needed as new issues and concerns arise.

The ethical principle of beneficence requires that potential benefits to individuals and to society be maximized and that potential harms be minimized [17]. Beneficence involves both the protection of individual welfare and the promotion of the common welfare. This principle underlies ethical rules and norms that require that public health institutions act in a timely manner on the information they have and that they expeditiously make the information available to the public [9]. The principle of nonmaleficence requires that harmful acts be avoided. However, the principle of nonmaleficence does not preclude balancing potential harms against potential benefits [14]. The principle of autonomy focuses on the right of self-determination. Respect for the individual is a principle rooted in the Western tradition, which grants importance to individual freedom in political life, and to personal development.

Principles of justice are also important [11, 13, 14]. Utilitarian theories of justice emphasize a mixture of criteria so that public utility is maximized. From this perspective, a just distribution of benefits from public health programs or research is determined by the utility to all affected. As noted by Childress et al. [8], public health activities are generally understood to be *consequentialist* in that the primary end that is sought is the health of the public. An egalitarian theory of justice holds that each person should share equally in the distribution of the potential benefits of health care resources such as screening services. Other theories of justice hold that society has an obligation to correct inequalities in the distribution of resources, and that those who are least well-off should benefit most from resources such as screening services. Such theories of justice provide considerable support for maximizing benefits to medically underserved people [13, 18].

Case-Based Approaches to Moral Reasoning

Although many general ethical questions have been answered on the basis of general principles and theories, the specific decisions that emerge in particular cases may remain unaddressed by the principles. Such decisions are often made by focusing on the circumstances of the case at hand and the moral context in which the case rests. Case-based methods such as casuistry are grounded in analogical reasoning, appeal to paradigmatic cases, and practical judgment [5, 14].

In casuistry, which in contemporary bioethics has been championed by Albert Jonsen and Stephen Toulmin [15, 19], decision-making takes place at the level of the particulars of the case itself. Given a case and a particular decision to be made, a casuist need not refer directly to a particular theory. Rather, maxims are identified that have bearing on the case. Maxims are wise, pithy, rule-like sayings such as "tell the truth" or "be compassionate."

Casuistry requires a clear exposition of the facts surrounding a case. A decision must then be made about which maxim is the most appropriate to "rule" or govern the case. Different circumstances or facts might call for a different maxim. A claim or judgment is then made regarding the case. The claim is backed by a form of logical reasoning described in terms of grounds or relevant circumstances, maxims, and the backings or more general notions that support the maxims. The descriptions of the case, including the circumstances, maxims, and logical thought, constitute its basic structure or morphology [14]. Placing a particular case alongside other similar cases has been referred to as taxonomy.

Casuistic reasoning begins with relatively clear, paradigmatic cases in which some ethical norm indicates the right course of action. Judgment is necessary to determine which norm applies in a complicated or ambiguous case.

Other Approaches to Moral Reasoning

Other approaches to moral reasoning, such as rights-based theories, duty-based theories, contractarianism, the ethics of care, narrative ethics, and communitarianism have not been widely applied in public health. Virtue ethics and the moral rule-based system of Gert and Clouser, however, have been discussed as potential alternatives to other leading approaches to moral reasoning in public health ethics [5, 20].

Moral disagreements can sometimes be resolved by obtaining further facts about matters at the center of the controversy or by defining more clearly the language used by the disputing parties [14]. Other steps that can be taken to resolve moral controversies include using examples and counterexamples and analyzing arguments to expose their inadequacies, gaps, and fallacies. In addition, moral problems can sometimes be resolved by getting the disputing parties to adopt a new policy or code, such as ethics guidelines for epidemiologists [14].

Ethical Issues in Epidemiology and Public Health Practice

The results of epidemiologic research studies contribute to generalizable knowledge by elucidating the causes of disease; by combining epidemiologic data with information from other disciplines such as genetics and microbiology; by evaluating the consistency of epidemiologic data with etiological hypotheses; and by providing the basis for developing and evaluating health promotion and prevention procedures [21]. The primary professional roles of epidemiology are the design and conduct of scientific research and the public health application of scientific knowledge. This includes reporting research results, and maintaining and promoting health in communities. In carrying out these professional roles, epidemiologists often encounter a number of ethical issues and concerns requiring careful consideration. Many of these issues have been addressed in the literature on ethics in epidemiology and public health practice including ethics guidelines.

Issues Dealt with in Ethics Guidelines for Epidemiologists and the Published Literature

Ethical and professional norms in epidemiology have been clarified in ethics guidelines for epidemiologists and other public health professionals [16, 22–24]. Ethics guidelines such as those developed for the Industrial Epidemiology Forum, the International Society for Environmental Epidemiology, and the American College of Epidemiology provide useful accounts of epidemiologists' obligations to research participants, society, employers, and colleagues. Ethics guidelines for environmental epidemiologists drafted by Colin Soskolne and Andrew Light [22], which were adopted by the International Society for Environmental Epidemiology in 1999, highlight the important obligations that epidemiologists have toward communities that are affected by environmental hazards. The ethics guidelines adopted by the American College of Epidemiology discuss core values, duties, and virtues in epidemiology; the professional role of epidemiologists; minimizing risks and protecting the welfare of research participants; providing benefits; ensuring an equitable distribution of risks and benefits; protecting confidentiality and privacy; obtaining informed consent; submitting proposed studies for ethical review; maintaining public trust; avoiding conflicts of interest and partiality; communicating ethical requirements; confronting unacceptable conduct; and obligations to communities [16]. International guidelines for ethical review of epidemiologic studies were published by the Council of International Organizations of Medical Sciences (CIOMS) [24]. The guidelines draw a distinction between epidemiologic research and routine practice (e.g., outbreak investigations and public health surveillance) and consider some of the issues associated with obtaining informed consent in epidemiologic studies. Specific ethical issues arising in epidemiologic research and public health practice that have been highlighted in ethics guidelines include minimizing risks and providing benefits, informed consent, avoiding and disclosing conflicts of interest, obligations to communities, and the institutional review board (IRB) system.

Minimizing Risks and Providing Benefits

Ethical concerns in epidemiology and public health practice often relate to the obligations of health professionals to acquire and apply scientific knowledge aimed at maintaining and restoring public health while respecting individual rights. Potential societal benefits must often be balanced with risks and potential harms to individuals and communities, such as the potential for stigmatization or invasions of privacy.

Epidemiologists have ethical and professional obligations to maximize the potential benefits of studies to research participants and to society, and to minimize potential harms and risks. In addition, these obligations are often legal or regulatory requirements, such as U.S. Federal regulations protecting human research participants [45 Code of Federal Regulations (CFR) 46]. The risks of epidemiologic studies and practice activities can be minimized by rigorously protecting the confidentiality of health information, as discussed below. Although the risks posed by epidemiologic studies are often minor compared with those that may be associated with clinical trials and other experimental studies, participants in epidemiologic studies may be burdened by a loss of privacy, by time spent completing interviews and examinations, and by possible adverse psychological effects such as enhanced grief or anxiety [25]. Such risks and potential harms can be minimized by careful attention to study procedures and questionnaire design, for example, by limiting the length of interviews or by scheduling them on a date that is less likely to result in adverse psychological effects.

Minimizing risks and potential harms and maximizing potential benefits are particularly important in epidemiologic studies on vulnerable populations. Examples include studies conducted on children, prisoners, some elderly people, and populations that are marginalized or socioeconomically disadvantaged.

A further obligation is the need to ensure that the burdens and potential benefits of epidemiologic studies are distributed equitably. The potential benefits of epidemiologic research are often societal in nature, such as obtaining new information about the causes of diseases, or identifying health disparities across groups defined by race, ethnicity, socioeconomic status, or other factors [25]. Research participants may receive direct benefits from participation in some studies, such as when a previously unrecognized disease or risk factor is detected during examinations. The balance of risks and potential benefits of epidemiologic studies are considered not only by individual researchers but also by members of human subjects committees such as IRBs in the United States.

Avoiding and Disclosing Conflicts of Interest

Other ethical issues that arise in the professional practice of epidemiology relate to how to best deal with potential conflicts of interest, in order to maintain public trust in epidemiology and sustain public support for health research. Recent media reports about previously undisclosed conflicts of interest in the United States and other countries have raised public awareness of the potential for conflicts of interest in clinical research and epidemiology, and about the need for institutions and individual researchers to address such conflicts. Conflicts of interest can affect scientific judgment and harm scientific objectivity. Studies have suggested that financial interests and researchers' commitment to a hypothesis can influence reported research results [26]. To address such concerns, funding agencies and research institutions have taken steps such as adopting new training programs that encourage researchers to avoid or disclose conflicts of interest, and revising or strengthening institutional rules and guidelines. Professional societies and medical associations have also issued policy statements and recommendations about how best to address conflicts of interest in clinical research [27]. Researchers should disclose financial interests and sources of funding when publishing research results. It may also be important to disclose information about potential or actual financial conflicts of interest when obtaining informed consent from research participants. A related issue is that health researchers should avoid entering into contractual agreements that prevent them from publishing results in a timely manner [16]. Communicating research results in a timely manner, without censorship or interference from the funder, is essential for maintaining public trust [9].

Obligations to Communities

The obligations of epidemiologists to study participants have been highlighted in several reports [16, 22]. These obligations include communicating the results of epidemiologic studies at the earliest possible time, after appropriate scientific peer review, so that the widest possible audience stands to benefit from the information. Epidemiologists should strive to carry out studies in a manner that is scientifically valid, and interpret and report the results of their studies in a manner that is scientifically accurate and appropriate. In addition, epidemiologists should respect cultural diversity in carrying out studies and in communicating with members of affected communities. Other obligations to community members and to research participants have been highlighted in ethics guidelines for epidemiologists and public health institutions [9].

Informed Consent

Informed consent provisions in public health studies ensure that research participants can make a free choice and also give institutions the legal authorization to proceed with the research [28]. Investigators must disclose information that potential participants use to decide whether to consent to the study. This includes the purpose of the research, the scientific procedures, anticipated risks and benefits, any inconveniences or discomfort, and the participant's right to refuse participation or to withdraw from the research at any time (45 CFR 46). Informed consent requirements may be waived in exceptional circumstances when obtaining consent is impractical, the risks are minimal, and the risks and potential benefits of the research have been carefully considered by an independent review committee. For example, in some epidemiology studies involving the analysis of large databases of routinely collected information (e.g., insurance claims data), it may not be feasible to recontact patients to ask them for their informed consent. Risks and potential harms in such studies may be very low, and risks may be further reduced by omitting personal identifiers from the computer databases.

Special considerations for obtaining informed consent may arise in public health studies of socioeconomically deprived people. People who have limited access to health care may misunderstand an invitation to participate in a study as an opportunity to receive medical care. In addition, they may be reluctant to refuse participation when the researcher is viewed as someone in a position of authority, such as a physician or university professor. Socioeconomically deprived people may also be more motivated to participate in studies involving financial incentives for participation. A further issue is that there is often a need to translate informed consent statements into a language other than English. The important issues arising in international research conducted by researchers from countries such as the United States and Great Britain in developing countries have also received considerable attention [24, 29].

Privacy and Confidentiality

One important way in which public health researchers reduce potential harms and risks to participants in epidemiologic studies is by rigorously protecting the confidentiality of their health information. Specific measures taken by researchers to protect the confidentiality of health information include keeping records under lock and key, limiting access to confidential records, discarding personal identifiers from data collection forms and computer files whenever feasible, and training staff in the importance of privacy and confidentiality protection [25]. Other measures that have been used to safeguard health information include encrypting computer databases, limiting geographic detail, and suppressing cells in tabulated data where the number of cases in the cell is small [30].

In the United States, the Health Insurance Portability and Accountability Act (HIPAA) of 1996 took effect early in 2004 after extensive planning and discussion [31]. The new regulations provide protection for the privacy of certain individually identifiable health data, referred to as protected health information. The privacy rules permit disclosures without individual authorization to public health authorities authorized by law to collect or receive the information for the purpose of preventing or controlling disease, injury, or disability, including public health practice activities such as surveillance.

The IRB System

The purpose of research ethics committees or IRBs is to ensure that studies involving human research participants are designed to conform with relevant ethical standards and that the rights and welfare of participants are protected. Human-subjects review by such committees ensures that studies have a favorable balance of potential benefits and risks, that participants are selected equitably, and that procedures for obtaining informed consent are adequate. In the United States, Federal regulations to protect human research subjects (45 CFR 46) have resulted in a complex IRB system. Similar safeguards exist in many other countries.

Despite the important role played by research ethics committees and IRBs, researchers have sometimes expressed concern about the obstacles that human-subjects review can create. In some countries, human-subjects review has been streamlined with the use of standardized forms and review processes or by centralizing review by research ethics committees [32]. As previously noted, one of the important issues considered by research ethics committees and by individual researchers is the adequacy of provisions for obtaining the informed consent of study participants.

These are just some of the ethical issues addressed in ethics guidelines developed for epidemiologists and other public health professionals. Other issues addressed in the guidelines include those pertaining to scientific misconduct, intellectual property and data sharing, publication of research findings, and cross-cultural or international health research.

Ethical Issues in Public Health Practice

An expanding body of literature has considered the important ethical issues that arise in such areas of public health practice as surveillance, emergency responses, and program evaluation [1, 4, 33–35]. In further specifying ethical norms in particular contexts, it is important to draw distinctions between epidemiologic research and public health practice activities. For example, requirements for submitting research protocols to an IRB do not necessarily apply to outbreak investigations and other emergency responses [36].

Definitions of Surveillance, Emergency Responses, and Program Evaluation

Surveillance can be defined as the ongoing, systematic collection, analysis, and interpretation of outcome-specific data, with the timely dissemination of these data to those responsible for preventing and controlling disease or injury [37]. A fundamental public health activity is to measure and monitor changes in health status, risk factors, and health service access and utilization. The effective dissemination of information is as important as data collection and analysis; the collected information must have a demonstrated utility [38].

Emergency responses and outbreak investigations can be defined as public health activities undertaken in an urgent or emergency situation, usually because of an imminent health threat to the population [39]. Sometimes this is because the public or government authorities perceive an imminent threat demanding immediate action. The primary purpose of the activity is to determine the nature and magnitude of a public health problem in the community and to implement appropriate measures to address the problem [39].

Field epidemiology and investigations of disease outbreaks require us to consider when the data are sufficient to take action rather than to ask what additional questions might be answered by the data [40]. The guidelines and approaches for conducting epidemiologic field investigations reflect the urgency of discovering causative factors and the need to make practical recommendations, such as during the severe acute respiratory syndrome epidemic [41]. Program evaluation, on the other hand, refers to the systematic application of scientific and statistical procedures for measuring program conceptualization, design, implementation, and utility; the comparison of these measurements; and the use of the resulting information to optimize program outcomes [36, 42, 43].

Federal regulations (Title 45 CFR Part 46), which deal with issues such as IRB review and informed consent requirements, mostly address biomedical research [36, 42, 43]. These regulations define research as a systematic investigation, including development, testing, and evaluation designed to develop or contribute to generalizable knowledge. Although some public health activities can clearly be classified as either research or nonresearch activities for regulatory purposes, for other activities the classification is more difficult. For example, scientific knowledge generated in controlling a disease outbreak may turn out to be useful in other settings, even though generating generalizable knowledge was not the primary intent of the investigation [36].

In applying the Federal regulations for protecting participants in public health research, U.S. agencies have distinguished health research and nonresearch public health practice activities. Research and nonresearch activities cannot be easily defined by the methods used. For example, questionnaire development, laboratory analysis, and logistic regression techniques are commonly used in etiologic studies with a case-control design, as well as in many case-control studies conducted as part of outbreak investigations. To address this issue, guidelines from the Centers for Disease Control and Prevention state that the major difference between research and nonresearch lies in the primary intent of the activity. The primary intent of research is to generate or contribute to generalizable knowledge. The primary intent of nonresearch activities in public health practice is to prevent disease or injury, improve health, and ensure the efficient and effective use of resources.

For example, surveillance projects are likely to be nonresearch when they involve the regular, ongoing collection and analysis of health-related data, conducted to monitor the frequency and distribution of diseases and health conditions in the population. Surveillance projects may have a research component when they involve the collection and analysis of health-related data conducted either to generate knowledge that is applicable to other populations and settings or to contribute to general knowledge about the health condition. Most emergency responses and outbreak investigations tend to be nonresearch because these projects are undertaken to solve an immediate health problem and any knowledge gained will likely benefit only the study participants or target population [36].

Although some ethical requirements, such as IRB review, do not apply equally to epidemiologic research and nonresearch public health practice activities, there are many important similarities between the ethics of epidemiologic research and nonresearch (e.g., requirements for confidentiality protection in research and nonresearch disease surveillance systems). Investigators should carefully consider ethical issues in each project, regardless of whether it is research or public health practice.

Ethical Issues in Public Health Surveillance

Ethics guidelines for public health surveillance have been developed for disease registry personnel, and a growing body of literature has evolved in this area, indicating increasing interest [4, 33–35, 44]. These developments are partly a response to public concern over the privacy and confidentiality of health information and technological advances such as the use of the Internet to disseminate data from surveillance systems and disease registries.

Data collected through surveillance systems provide for the ongoing evaluation of disease risk factors, incidence, and mortality, and allow for the evaluation of health care utilization, treatment, and disease prevention and control activities [45]. These and other benefits of public health surveillance must be balanced against possible risks and harms, such as infringements on personal privacy. The need to balance potential benefits against risks underlines the rule that surveillance data should not be collected if they will not be used [44]. Thus, public health professionals have ethical obligations to both maximize the potential benefits of routinely collected surveillance and disease registry data and minimize risks and potential harms. Steps taken to assure the quality of data collected by public health surveillance systems and disease registries maximize the potential benefits of the data. Registry data must be accurate, complete, and timely.

Potential harms and risks from the collection and use of surveillance and registry data include loss of privacy and harms resulting from breaches of confidentiality. These risks are remote possibilities because of the steps taken by public health professionals to safeguard the confidentiality of personally identifiable records in surveillance systems and registries, such as data encryption, written policies and procedures for confidentiality and disclosure of data, and training of staff.

The privacy rules included in HIPAA permit disclosures without individual authorization to public health authorities who can legally collect or receive the information for the purpose of preventing or controlling disease, injury, or disability. This includes public health practice activities such as surveillance.

Health Promotion and Disease Prevention

The potential benefits of disease prevention and health promotion efforts include a healthier society and reduced fiscal expenditure and increased productivity and efficiency [46]. Individual members of society can also benefit. There is a need to balance health as a value with values of privacy and autonomy (e.g., in relation to immunization policies). Several authors have considered the circumstances under which personal autonomy can be abridged to promote the health of the whole community and the moral justification for coercive public health interventions and lifestyle strategies [47, 48]. As noted by Lappé [1], "From an ethical perspective, the extent to which [compulsive public health] interventions are justified depends on . . . the anticipated extent and kind of public benefit; the degree to which individual rights are restricted to achieve that benefit; and the ultimate distribution of both benefits and harms attendant to participation."

In general, there is a need for voluntariness in health education, health promotion, and public health communication programs. The risks and potential harms of public health interventions include ineffective, counterproductive, or harmful interventions; unanticipated consequences; and labeling or stigmatizing of individuals [49]. Undue stress on the individual's role in the cause of illness could lead to a "blame the victim" mentality [48]. The dilemma is how to advise people that they might be at risk for potentially serious health complications without labeling them, contributing to their anxiety, or adversely affecting their well-being [49].

Ethical considerations for prevention trials and community interventions include an assessment of risks and benefits, the need for voluntary participation and avoidance of excessive incentives, and justice-related issues. There is a need for sensitivity to ethnic and cultural habits and norms and to avoid "top-down" planning, in which the health concerns and self-defined information needs of the target population are ignored in favor of professional preoccupations and concerns. Such concerns have been successfully addressed through community-based participatory research, which is a collaborative, empowering process that helps develop competencies in communities [50]. Ethical issues in health communication include the need to avoid conflicts of interest, to present facts about health hazards or health opportunities in a truthful, balanced, and timely fashion, and to avoid distorting the facts or concealing ambiguities in the scientific evidence [49].

Ethical Issues in Screening

Ethical issues also arise in public health screening programs [51]. Screening is the presumptive identification of an unrecognized disease or condition by the use of tests, examinations, or other procedures that can help identify a disease or disease precursor in apparently healthy people. People with positive or suspicious findings subsequently undergo further evaluation or treatment. The ultimate objective of screening is to reduce the morbidity or mortality from a disease among the people screened.

Several frameworks for analyzing and addressing ethical and policy issues in public health screening programs have been proposed. In 1968, Wilson and Jungner [52] proposed 10 principles for mass screening programs. These principles are often cited in planning and evaluating population screening programs; they relate to the adequacy of the scientific evidence, the balance of risks and benefits, the availability of an effective treatment, the acceptability of the screening test to the population, and the costs and resources required [51]. Refinements have been proposed over the years, with further specification of the principles of screening [53–56]. Criteria for the effectiveness of clinical preventive services have been developed by the Canadian Task Force on the Periodic Health Examination [57] and by the U.S. Preventive Services Task Force [58]. Screening raises a number of important ethical issues around informed consent, privacy and confidentiality, risks and potential benefits, and the allocation of finite public resources for screening.

The principle of respect for individuals' freedom supports the right of participants to informed consent before screening [51]. Provisions for informed consent ensure that people undergoing screening make free choices, and encourage providers to act responsibly in their interactions with patients. Subjects should be given information about the procedure, the meaning of a positive or negative test result, and any appreciable risks or potential harms and benefits before undergoing screening [51]. To give informed consent for screening, participants need to understand the risk of a false positive test result and the procedures that may follow it [59].

Principles of informed consent for screening have some features in common with emerging models of informed decision-making and shared decision-making for screening and other health care services [60]. Such models emphasize that people should be provided with balanced and relevant information so they can make informed decisions about screening options [61–63]. As discussed by Briss et al. [62], informed decision-making occurs when the participant understands the nature of the disease or condition being addressed; understands the clinical service and its likely consequences, including risks, limitations, benefits, alternatives, and uncertainties; has considered his or her preferences as appropriate; has participated in decision-making at a personally desirable level; and either makes a decision consistent with his or her preferences and values or elects to defer a decision to a later time.

Although public health screening is generally voluntary, some examples of mandatory screening can be cited. For example, most states require that infants be screened for certain genetic disorders, such as phenylketonuria. Infants are subject to the screening program unless their parents refuse for religious or philosophical reasons [51]. Public health officials may justify mandatory newborn screening programs, even without parental consent, under utilitarian principles authorizing state governments to protect children [51].

The potential benefits of screening include the early detection of disease and the prevention of serious illness or disability and improved survival. The societal benefits of screening include substantial reductions in morbidity and mortality [58]. Screening is undertaken for conditions that are important public health problems and those for which early detection and treatment are effective. If early treatment is not effective, then early detection alone merely extends the length of time the disease is known to exist, without extending survival [59]. Public health policymakers rely on information from randomized controlled trials and other sources to evaluate the effectiveness, potential benefits, and risks or potential harms of screening.

The potential harms and risks associated with screening also have to be taken into account, especially since screening programs are aimed at large numbers of apparently healthy people. Minor complications or infrequent adverse effects that would be acceptable in the treatment of a severe illness take on greater importance when screening asymptomatic people and require careful evaluation to determine whether the potential benefits exceed risks [58]. There may be risks associated with false positive or false negative test results. The potential harms of screening may also include "labeling" effects and the psychological impact of test results or a diagnosis. If prognosis is not improved by presymptomatic detection, screening for a disease can cause anxiety without providing any benefit [56]. Medical information collected as part of screening should be rigorously safeguarded to protect patient privacy and confidentiality and to minimize risks or potential harms such as stigma or discrimination. Only a few specific exceptions exist, such as mandatory partner notification laws for human immunodeficiency virus infection that physicians are legally required to follow in some states [64].

Summary and Conclusions

The burgeoning interest in ethical issues in epidemiologic research and public health practice reflects both the important societal role of public health and the growing public interest in the scientific integrity of health information and the equitable distribution of health care resources. Attention to ethical issues can facilitate the effective planning, implementation, and growth of a variety of public health programs and research activities. Seen from this perspective, public health ethics is consistent with the prevention orientation of public health. Ethical concerns can be anticipated or identified early and effectively addressed through careful analysis and consultation.

Acknowledgments

The findings and conclusions in this article are those of the author and do not necessarily represent the official position of the Centers for Disease Control and Prevention.

References

1. Lappé, M. Ethics and Public Health. In: Last, J.M., editor, *Maxcy–Rosenau's Public Health and Preventive Medicine* (12th ed.). Norwalk, CT: Appleton-Century-Crofts (1986):1867–1877.
2. Soskolne, C.L. Rationalizing Professional Conduct: Ethics in Disease Control. *Public Health Rev* (1991):19:311–321.
3. Coughlin, S.S., and T.L. Beauchamp. Historical Foundations. In: *Ethics and Epidemiology.* New York, NY: Oxford University Press (1996):5–23.
4. Coughlin, S.S. Ethics in Epidemiology and Public Health Practice. In: *Ethics in Epidemiology and Public Health Practice: Collected Works.* Columbus, GA: Quill Publications (1997):9–26.
5. Coughlin, S.S., C.L. Soskolne, and K.W. Goodman. Case Analysis and Moral Reasoning. In: *Case Studies in Public Health Ethics.* Washington, D.C.: American Public Health Association (1997):1–18.
6. Beauchamp, D.E., and B. Steinbock, editors. *New Ethics for the Public's Health.* New York, NY: Oxford University Press (1999).
7. Callahan, D., and B. Jennings. Ethics and Public Health: Forging a Strong Relationship. *Am J Public Health* (2002):92:169–176.
8. Childress, J.F., R.R. Faden, R.D. Gaare, L.O. Gostin, J. Kahn, R.J. Bonnie, N.E. Kass, A.C. Mastroianni, J.D. Moreno, and P. Nieburg. Public Health Ethics: Mapping the Terrain. *J Law Med Ethics* (2002):30:170–178.
9. Public Health Leadership Society. Principles of the Ethical Practice of Public Health, 2000 (available at http://www.phls.org). (Also adopted by the American Public Health Association and available at http://www.apha.org/codeofethics/ethics.htm).
10. Bayer, R., and A.L. Fairchild. The Genesis of Public Health Ethics. *Bioethics* (2004):18:473–492.
11. Kass, N.E. Public Health Ethics: from Foundations and Frameworks to Justice and Global Public Health. *J Law Med Ethics* (2004):32:232–242.
12. Coughlin, S.S. Model Curricula in Public Health Ethics. *Am J Prev Med* (1996):12:247–251.
13. Anand, S., F. Peter, and A. Sen. *Public Health, Ethics, and Equity.* New York, NY: Oxford University Press (2004).
14. Beauchamp, T.L. Moral Foundations. In: Coughlin, S.S., and T.L. Beauchamp, editors, *Ethics and Epidemiology.* New York, NY: Oxford University Press (1996):24–52.
15. Jonsen, A.R., and S.E. Toulmin. *The Abuse of Casuistry.* Berkeley, CA: University of California Press (1988).
16. American College of Epidemiology. Ethics Guidelines. *Ann Epidemiol* (2000):10:487–497.
17. Beauchamp, T.L., and J.F. Childress. *Principles of Biomedical Ethics* (4th ed.). New York, NY: Oxford University Press (1996).
18. Powers, M., and R. Faden. *Social Justice: The Moral Foundations of Public Health and Health Policy.* New York, NY: Oxford University Press (2006).
19. Jonsen, A.R. Casuistry: An Alternative or Complement to Principles? *Kennedy Inst Ethics* (1995):5:237–251.

20. Weed, D.L., and R.E. McKeown. Epidemiology and Virtue Ethics. *Int J Epidemiol* (1998):27:343–348.

21. Lilienfeld, A.M., and D.E. Lilienfeld. *Foundations of Epidemiology* (2nd ed.). New York, NY: Oxford University Press (1980).

22. Soskolne, C.L., and A. Light. Towards Ethics Guidelines for Environmental Epidemiologists. *Sci Total Environ* (1996):184:137–147.

23. Beauchamp, T.L., R.R. Cook, and W.E. Fayerweather. Ethical Guidelines for Epidemiologists. *J Clin Epidemiol* (1991):44(I Suppl):151S–169S.

24. Council for International Organizations of Medical Sciences. International Guidelines for Ethical Review of Epidemiological Studies. *Law Med Health Care* (1991):19:247–258.

25. Coughlin, S.S. Ethically Optimized Study Designs in Epidemiology. In: Coughlin, S.S., and T.L. Beauchamp, editors, *Ethics and Epidemiology*. New York, NY: Oxford University Press (1996):145–55.

26. Seigel, D. Clinical Trials, Epidemiology, and Public Confidence. *Stat Med* (2003):22:3419–3425.

27. AAMC Task Force on Financial Conflicts of Interest in Clinical Research. Protecting Subjects, Preserving Trust, Promoting Progress: II. Principles and Recommendations for Oversight of an Institution's Financial Interests in Human Subjects Research. *Acad Med* (2003):78:237–245.

28. Shulz, M. Legal and Ethical Considerations in Securing Consent to Epidemiologic Research in the United States. In: Coughlin, S.S., and T.L. Beauchamp, editors, *Ethics and Epidemiology*. New York, NY: Oxford University Press (1996):97–127.

29. Macklin, R. *Against Relativism: Cultural Diversity and the Search for Ethical Universals in Medicine*. New York, NY: Oxford University Press (1999).

30. Wynia, M.K., S.S. Coughlin, S. Alpert, D.S. Cummins, and L.L. Emanuel. Shared Expectations for Protection of Identifiable Health Care Information. Report of a National Consensus Process. *J Gen Intern Med* (2001):16:100–111.

31. Centers for Disease Control and Prevention. HIPAA Privacy Rule and Public Health. Guidance from CDC and the U.S. Department of Health and Human Services. *MMWR* (2003):52:1–12.

32. Pattison, J., and T. Stacey. Research Bureaucracy in the United Kingdom. *BMJ* (2004):329:622–624.

33. Hahn, R.A. Ethical Issues. In: Teutsch, S.M. and R.E. Churchill, editors, *Principles and Practice of Public Health Surveillance*. New York, NY: Oxford University Press (1994):175–89.

34. Gostin, L.O. Health Information: Reconciling Personal Privacy with the Public Good of Human Health. *Health Care Anal* (2001):9:321–335.

35. Fairchild, A.L., and R. Bayer. Ethics and the Conduct of Public Health Surveillance. *Science* (2004):303:631–632.

36. Snider, D.E., and D.F. Stroup. Defining Research When It Comes to Public Health. *Public Health Rep* (1997):112:29–112.

37. Thacker, S.B., and R.L. Berkelman. Public Health Surveillance in the United States. *Epidemiol Rev* (1988):10:164–190.

38. Wetterhall, S.F., M. Pappaioanou, and S.B. Thacker. The Role of Public Health Surveillance: Information for Effective Action in Public Health. *MMWR* (1992):41(Suppl):207–218.

39. Langmuir, A.D. The Epidemic Intelligence Service of the Centers for Disease Control. *Public Health Rep* (1980):95:470–477.

40. Goodman, R.A., and J.W. Buehler. Field Epidemiology Defined. In: Gregg, M.B., R.C. Dicker, and R.A. Goodman, editors, *Field Epidemiology*. New York, NY: Oxford University Press (1996):3–7.

41. Singer, P.A., S.R. Benatar, M. Bernstein, A.S. Daar, B.M. Dickens, S.K. MacRae, R.E.G. Upshur, L. Wright, and R.Z. Shaul. Ethics and SARS: Lessons from Toronto. *BMJ* (2003):327:1342–1344.

42. Rossi, P.H., and H.E. Freeman. *Evaluation: A Systematic Approach*. Newbury Park, CA: Sage Publications (1993).
43. Centers for Disease Control and Prevention. Framework for Program Evaluation in Public Health. *MMWR* (1999):48(RR11):1–40.
44. Coughlin, S.S., G.G. Clutter, and M. Hutton. Ethics in Cancer Registries. *J Registry Manag* (1999):5–10.
45. Chen, V.W. The Right to Know vs. the Right to Privacy. *J Registry Manag* (1997):27(4):125–127.
46. Pellegrino, E.D. Autonomy and Coercion in Disease Prevention and Health Promotion. *Theor Med* (1984):5:83–91.
47. Faden, R.R. Ethical Issues in Government Sponsored Public Health Campaigns. *Health Educ Q* (1987):14:27–37.
48. Wikler, D.I. Persuasion and Coercion for Health. *Milbank Mem Fund Q* (1978):56:303–338.
49. Guttman, N. Ethical Dilemmas in Health Campaigns. *Health Commun* (1997):9:155–190.
50. Glanz, K., B.K. Rimer, and C. Lerman. Ethical Issues in the Design and Conduct of Community-Based Intervention Studies. In: Coughlin, S.S. and T.L. Beauchamp, editors, *Ethics and Epidemiology*. New York, NY: Oxford University Press (1996).
51. Burke, W., S.S. Coughlin, N.C. Lee, D. Weed, and M. Khoury. Application of Population Screening Principles to Genetic Screening for Adult-Onset Conditions. *Genet Test* (2001):5:201–11.
52. Wilson, J.M.G., and F. Jungner. *Principles and Practice of Screening for Disease*. Public Health Papers No. 34. Geneva: World Health Organization (1968).
53. Cadman, D., L. Chambers, W. Feldman, and D. Sackett. Assessing the Effectiveness of Community Screening Programs. *JAMA* (1984):251:1580–1585.
54. Miller, A.B. Principles of Screening and of the Evaluation of Screening Programs. In: Miller, A.B., editor, *Screening for Cancer*. San Diego, CA: Academic Press (1985):3–24.
55. Cole, P., and A.S. Morrison. Basic Issues in Population Screening for Cancer. *J Natl Cancer Inst* (1980):64:1263–1272.
56. Sox, H.C. Preventive Health Services in Adults. *N Engl J Med* (1994):330:1589–1595.
57. Canadian Task Force on the Periodic Health Examination. *Canadian Guide to Clinical Preventive Health Care*. Ottawa: Canada Communication Group (1994).
58. U.S. Preventive Services Task Force. *Guide to Clinical Preventive Services*. Baltimore, MD: Lippincott Williams and Wilkins (1996).
59. Lee, J.M. Screening and Informed Consent. *N Engl J Med* (1993):328:438–440.
60. Whitney, S.N., A.L. McGuire, and L.B. McCullogh. A Typology of Shared Decision Making, Informed Consent, and Simple Consent. *Ann Intern Med* (2003):140:54–59.
61. Hewitson, P., and J. Austoker. Patient Information, Informed Decision-Making, and the Psycho-Social Impact of Prostate-Specific Antigen Testing. *BJU Int* (2005):95(3 Suppl):16–32.
62. Briss, P., B. Rimer, B. Reilley, R.C. Coates, N.C. Lee, P. Mullen, P. Corso, A.B. Hutchinson, R. Hiatt, J. Kerner, P. George, C. White, N. Gandhi, M. Saraiya, R. Breslow, G. Isham, S.M. Teutsch, A.R. Hinman, and R. Lawrence. Promoting Informed Decisions about Cancer Screening in Communities and Healthcare Systems. *Am J Prev Med* (2004):26:67–80.
63. Sheridan, S.L., R.P. Harris, and S.H. Woolf. Shared Decision Making about Screening and Chemoprevention. A Suggested Approach from the U.S. Preventive Services Task Force. *Am J Prev Med* (2004):26:56–66.
64. Khalsa, A.M. Preventive Counseling, Screening, and Therapy for the Patient with Newly Diagnosed HIV Infection. *Am Fam Physician* (2006):15:271–280.

CHAPTER 6

ETHICS IN CANCER REGISTRIES

S.S. Coughlin, G.G. Clutter, and M. Hutton

There has been increasing interest in the ethics of cancer registration as shown by renewed emphasis on codes of ethics and ethics guidelines for cancer registry professionals, presentations on confidentiality and privacy protection at national and international meetings, and the burgeoning literature in this area [1–8]. These developments have been prompted, in part, by public concern over the privacy and confidentiality of health information, proposed restrictions in some countries on the use of medical records for disease surveillance and research purposes, and technological advances such as the use of the Internet to disseminate cancer registry data [6, 9–11].

Codes of ethics and ethics guidelines developed for cancer registry professionals identify core values and specific ethical norms that are widely held and accepted in the field [1, 2]. Sound judgment and reflection upon the core values and ethical rules described in the codes and guidelines are required for ethical decision-making.

This paper examines some of the important ethical precepts in the cancer registry profession, including those described in codes of ethics and ethics guidelines that have been developed for cancer registrars and other professionals who work in cancer registration. Topics include provisions for maximizing the societal benefits of cancer registries and minimizing risks and potential harms to patients, requirements for protecting confidentiality and privacy, responding to requests for use of registry data, and measures for maintaining public trust. Maintaining public trust consists of avoiding conflicts of interest, communicating ethical requirements for colleagues, and confronting unacceptable conduct. Cancer registry professionals such as cancer registrars and epidemiologists should be well informed about these topics because they are central to the maintenance and utilization of cancer registry data; in addition, recent developments may impact on local, regional, and national registries. Although this paper focuses on cancer registration, the issues examined also apply to other disease registries. We begin with some examples of ethical concerns of cancer registry professionals in order to provide a basis for the discussion of ethical norms and values that follows.

Examples of Ethical Concerns of Cancer Registry Professionals

First case. A state medical association sponsored a bill in the legislature to amend the current cancer registry statute. The bill would have required that contact with reported cancer patients for research purposes be made only with the patient's prior consent. Obtaining consent would require a written request to the managing physician, asking him or her to forward the request to the patient. Other groups, including the state cancer

"Ethics in Cancer Registries" originally appeared in the Journal of Registry Management (1999):26:5–10. Used with permission of the National Cancer Registrars Association's Journal of Registry Management.

registrars association, were against the proposed legislation because it would have hampered legitimate research. (This first case deals with the issue of whether prior consent should be required to recontact cancer patients identified through a registry to potentially include them in a research study, but disputes have arisen in other states over the even more controversial issue of whether prior consent should be required to include information about patients in a disease surveillance registry [11]). Agreement was eventually reached (which will require modification of the registry regulations) on a procedure by which patients will be notified of their registration in the state registry, and of the possibility of their being invited to take part in research studies.

Second case. Coal tar left in underground tanks was blamed for cases of childhood cancer in a small town in the United States [12]. The children and their parents sued a public service company and an engineering firm. The state department of public health was served with a subpoena demanding that files containing health information be turned over to the court. The following year, the director of the department of public health was served with a related subpoena demanding an exhaustive list of documents relating to the department's childhood cancer data. The department and its officers responded that the documents were privileged health data and that maintaining the confidentiality of the data was essential. A circuit court ordered the department to produce the cancer registry data by listing the type of cancer, date of diagnosis, and zip code for each cancer patient [12].

Third case. Members of the National Cancer Registrars Association (NCRA) ethics committee published an article in the association's newsletter explaining the obligations of cancer registrars to maintain the integrity of the profession, and their responsibility to protect the organization and its members [13]. A case scenario was provided with study questions to illustrate how a cancer registrar should respond to an apparent violation of the association's code of ethics by a coworker. It was emphasized that "whenever an allegation is made, there should always be supporting documentation. . . . The complaint should not be frivolous, and all registrars should maintain high standards of conduct, integrity, and fairness in all their professional actions and decisions" [13].

Core Values and the Professional Role of Cancer Registry Professionals

The ethics codes and guidelines developed by the NCRA and the International Association of Cancer Registries (IACR) discuss core values in the cancer registry profession as well as specific ethical rules and norms [1, 2]. Core values are fundamental ethical and scientific precepts, that is, basic scientific values, that underlie the mission and purpose of the field—for example, the need to develop, use, and maintain hospital-based or centralized cancer registries that meet the needs of physicians, administrators, planners, and researchers in reducing morbidity and mortality from cancer, while protecting individuals' rights to privacy and meeting other ethical and professional obligations [1]. Core values that are internal to the profession are more restricted in scope than general ethical principles such as those identified in the report of the National Commission on Biomedical and Behavioral Research (the Belmont Report) [14] and in recent frameworks for public health ethics [12, 15].

The professional role of cancer registrars has been identified in codes of ethics and in other documents [1–5, 16]. Cancer registrars significantly contribute to the collection of data on the occurrence of cancer in the population, and provide an important resource for clinical and epidemiological research [2]. The data they collect provide a basis for evaluating treatment modalities and patient survival, determining cancer incidence in defined populations, identifying high-risk groups for targeted cancer prevention and control activities, and assisting in the evaluation of prevention and control activities [3]. Cooperation and collaboration with other health professionals are an important part of the professional role of cancer registrars. For example, the NCRA code of ethics [1] states: "Cooperation with other professions and entities engaged in or supportive of health services is an essential factor in the cancer registry profession's greater aim of improving health services and supporting research relevant to the advancement of medical care."

Ethical Obligations of Cancer Registry Professionals

With these definitions and clarifications in mind, we now turn to a discussion of some of the major ethical obligations of cancer registrars and other cancer registry professionals, including the duty to maximize benefits and minimize risks.

Maximizing Benefits

Cancer registry professionals have ethical obligations to maximize the potential benefits of routinely collected data, to minimize risks, and to avoid causing harm [1, 2, 17–20]. They should evaluate the long-term benefits and risks that may result from increased knowledge and medical developments. A further obligation is to ensure that the potential benefits of cancer registries are distributed equitably [17]. For example, the need to balance potential benefits against risks to patients underlies the rule that surveillance data should not be collected if they will not be used. Of course, these obligations are not the sole responsibility of cancer registrars; members of institutional review boards (IRBs) and groups of investigators have similar responsibilities.

As an example of how the potential benefits of surveillance systems can be maximized, cancer registry data in some states are reported periodically by only two or three racial categories, for example, white, black, and other. The stratification and reporting of such routinely collected data into other racial categories (e.g., Native Americans) can provide important information about cancer mortality among population subgroups, and assist in targeting prevention and control efforts [17]. However, care must be taken to avoid inadvertently identifying individuals by reporting information about small numbers of cases.

Cancer registrars play an important role in maximizing the benefits of cancer registry data by assuring that data are of the highest quality [1, 21, 22]. Incorrect conclusions may be drawn from analyses of low-quality data, and that could potentially impair patient care or result in the misdirection of resources. A registrar has access to detailed information contained in a patient's medical record. He or she is responsible for its accurate translation into a case abstract. Sufficient attention to detail and appropriate consultation of manuals (especially for a complicated case) depend on the registrar's sound judgment. Decisions that are made at the point of case abstraction ultimately determine the quality of cancer data. Coding may or may not take into account all of the available information. Sometimes, only the registrar will know if a specific piece of information was considered while coding a given case. In such areas of uncertainty, professional ethics and standards of practice come into play. Professional ethics do not dictate exactly how much time should be spent in tracking down the details of a difficult case; instead, ethics standards help the registrar to understand that accurate and complete data provide benefits that justify the risks and potential harms of cancer registration, such as loss of privacy. From this perspective,

Table 6.1 Beneficial Uses of Local and Central Cancer Registry Data

Central Cancer Registries

Uses of central cancer registry data that provide potential benefits include:

- Detecting potential public health problems, for example, elevated cancer rates

- Identifying regional or national patterns of cancer risk

- Informing health professionals and the general public about risks, early detection, and treatment of cancer in the community

- Assisting in the identification and investigation of cancer clusters

- Providing information to address public concerns and questions about cancer

- Targeting cancer control intervention resources

- Providing data to qualified researchers for clinical or epidemiologic research into the causes of cancer

- Providing data to evaluate the cost, quality, efficacy, and appropriateness of diagnostic, therapeutic, rehabilitative, and preventive services and programs relating to cancer

Local Cancer Registries

Local cancer registry data can be used for the following:

- The administrative planning and allocation of hospital resources enabling health care institutions to provide cost-effective services to the community

- Treatment, planning, staging, and continuity of care for cancer patients

- Continuous medical surveillance and end-results reporting (survival analysis) to evaluate the effectiveness of diagnostic and treatment modalities used

- Continuous monitoring of health care facility results through quality measurement activities

- The evaluation of the accessibility and availability of health care services

- The evaluation of the appropriateness of services provided, the absence of clinically unnecessary diagnostic or therapeutic procedures, and the likelihood of favorable outcomes

Table 6.1 (*continued*)

- The evaluation of practitioner and support staff performance to assure appropriate and timely consultation, diagnosis, follow-up, and referrals as well as assessment of the need for interventions aimed at improving performance

- The monitoring and documentation of the appropriateness, accuracy, and completeness of clinical care provided to ensure that diagnosis and treatment are consistent with current professional knowledge

- The provision of data to central and other regional cancer registries to be used in research studies and for the calculation of population based rates

- The provision of data to the American College of Surgeons National Cancer Data Base to allow for comparisons between local, regional, and national trends in management and survival and to establish national standards in cancer patient care

the registrar can make a sound decision about how much time to spend tracking down and coding details of even a difficult case. Both the American College of Surgeons and the North American Association of Central Cancer Registries have published standards for quality assurance procedures for registry data [21, 22]. However, the rigor with which these standards are applied is often an individual decision guided by professional ethics.

Cancer registry data have several potentially beneficial uses (Table 6.1). One potential use relates to the efficient allocation of limited resources to provide maximum benefits to communities. Determining appropriate resource allocation may be achieved by identifying services that are most needed in specific populations through the evaluation of the accessibility and availability of health care services [3, 4]. This can allow for the targeting of intervention programs such as mammography screening in a particular geographic area or among underserved members of a community.

Cancer registry data may also be used to monitor the quality, efficacy, and appropriateness of cancer services at a health care facility or in the community [3, 4]. Cancer services in a community or region can be compared with local, regional, or national data, including trends in cancer services. One example is the evaluation of the use of radiation therapy following lumpectomy for breast cancer by comparing regional differences in the use of this procedure. Other examples are national or regional comparisons of stage-at-cancer diagnosis or survival rates.

Another potential benefit is the use of data to determine the need for cancer education programs for the general public or for continuing professional education. For example, if a community has an increased incidence of late-stage disease for a particular cancer site, patients may be slow to seek health care evaluation, or physicians may not be making the diagnosis soon enough. Professional or community education programs can then be tailored to meet the specific needs of the community.

Minimizing Risks

Potential harms and risks from the collection and utilization of cancer registry data include loss of privacy and loss of employment or insurance resulting from breaches of confidentiality [10, 19, 20]. These risks are admittedly remote possibilities because of the steps taken by cancer registrars to safeguard the confidentiality of personally identifiable records [1, 2, 5, 21]. Such problems are even less likely to occur with surveillance system data in which personal identifiers are intentionally omitted or discarded [17, 18].

Protecting Confidentiality and Privacy

Another important ethical obligation of cancer registry professionals is to protect the confidentiality and privacy of health information [1–8, 21]. As Clive and Miller [16] explained, "Cancer registrars are the trustees of cancer information, ensuring its accuracy, completeness, and timely reporting while at the same time protecting the privacy of the cancer patients." The ethical and legal obligations of cancer registry professionals to rigorously protect patient privacy and the confidentiality of health information have been discussed in several reviews [3, 5] and in ethics codes and guidelines developed by the NCRA, the North American Association of Central Cancer Registries (NAACCR), and the IACR [1, 2, 21]. These issues have again moved to the forefront because of public concern over computerized records and loss of privacy, newly enacted or proposed state laws, the Health Insurance Portability and Accountability Act of 1996, and proposed legislation in the United States and other countries [6, 11, 23]. The Health Insurance Portability and Accountability Act of 1996 includes provisions for privacy and security standards for individually identifiable health care information, with the goal of encouraging the development of a uniform health information system and increasing the efficiency of the health care system [23].

The dissemination of cancer registry data via the Internet, which facilitates their use by local communities and states to plan cancer prevention and control programs, has also raised new confidentiality concerns [10, 20]. An increasing number of public use data sets are being placed on the Internet to maximize the public health benefits by disseminating the information as widely as possible. However, even when personal identifiers are removed from such data sets, patients may be reidentified through data linkages [24]. Steps that can be taken to address such concerns are being considered by NAACCR members and sponsoring organizations [25].

The NAACCR Standards for Cancer Registries [21] define confidential data as patient-specific data that could identify a particular patient as well as "any information that specifically identifies a health care professional or an institution." As discussed by Muir and Demaret [5], the purpose of confidentiality measures in cancer registration is twofold: (1) to ensure the anonymity of individuals reported to the registry and, if necessary, for those making such notifications; and (2) to ensure that the best usage of cancer registry data is for the benefit of the cancer patient, for cancer control, and for medical research.

The NCRA Code of Ethics directly addresses confidentiality concerns [1]. Section I, Part A, calls for cancer registrars to "Uphold the doctrine of confidentiality and the individual's right to privacy in the disclosure of personally identifiable medical and social information." Other confidentiality-related principles in the NCRA Code of Ethics (Section I, Part A) include: "Use and release of identifiable and nonidentifiable information shall be according to the established institutional policies . . . every effort must be made to ensure that the computerization of cancer registry information is accomplished in a manner that protects the confidentiality of patient information."

Confidentiality issues in cancer registration have also been addressed by the NAACCR and the IACR [2, 21]. Their guidelines and standards for cancer registries are of particular interest to those who work in central cancer registries. The NAACCR standards, for example, include standards for confidentiality and disclosure of data and confidentiality policies and procedures relating to data collection and management [21]. These policies and procedures include the registry's responsibilities to protect its data from unauthorized access and release, standards for policies and procedures for data security, and standards for policies and procedures for release of registry data.

The IACR Guidelines on Confidentiality in the Cancer Registry [2] explain how confidentiality safeguards protect the right to privacy: "Guidelines for the maintenance of confidentiality are needed primarily to provide adequate safeguards for the individual's right to privacy, so that identifiable information on persons registered with cancer does not reach unauthorized third parties, while at the same time preserving the right of the individual, and that of his or her fellow citizens, to benefit from the knowledge on cancer causation, prevention, treatment, and survival that can be obtained from cancer registration and research."

The IACR Guidelines on Confidentiality provide a definition of confidential data similar to the one provided by the NAACCR, and enumerate several principles of confidentiality [2]. These principles include issues regarding the sharing of confidential clinical information, the scope of confidentiality measures, issues surrounding indirectly identifiable data, and methods of data storage and transmission. The confidentiality of data on deceased persons is also discussed in the IACR guidelines [2].

Specific steps that are taken by investigators to protect privacy and confidentiality in registry-based epidemiologic studies include keeping records with personal identifiers under lock and key, limiting access to confidential records on a need-to-know basis, discarding personal identifiers from forms and computer files whenever feasible, and reinforcing the importance of maintaining the confidentiality of health records at the time of orientation and training sessions for staff. In addition, results are released only in aggregated form to prevent breaches of confidentiality [10, 17, 26].

Responding to Requests for Data

The potential benefits of a registry can only be maximized if the data are used [3]. However, the release of data can pose risks. It is often the registrar's responsibility to decide what data to release and to whom. The institution's written policies and procedures for data release guide the registrar, but may not cover every situation. Professional norms and ethics, especially the need to maximize benefits while minimizing risks and protecting the patient's right to privacy, can guide the registrar when responding to requests for data.

When responding to requests for data, a registrar might consider the following issues:

- The institution's policies and procedures with regard to release of information. Every institution should have these available [8, 22] and the registrar should be knowledgeable about them.

- The proposed use of the data and whether it is an approved use according to written policies.
- Whether the available data can meet the purpose of the request. For example, if a researcher wants to study benign brain tumors or nonmelanoma skin cancer and such information is not routinely collected by the registry, the requestor should be notified.
- The amount and content of data that will meet the needs of the requestor while minimizing the risk of violating the patient's right to privacy. In general, data released should only be as specific and complete as is needed to answer a request by a qualified individual.
- Data format of information to be provided to requestor. For example, data could be released as aggregate tables, in the form of a report with charts and graphs, or as individual records. Information could be provided electronically or in hard copy.
- The amount and content of data that are released. For example, all the data in the database could be provided or summarized, or only data on certain cancers, from a certain period, or from specific fields may be provided. In addition, the data could be released with or without personal identifiers. The Commission on Cancer requires that requests for data that identify individual patients or physicians be reviewed by the cancer committee [27].
- Requestor's knowledge of confidentiality rules/procedures. Sometimes a registrar may need to educate an inexperienced researcher on the institution's rules for protecting patient confidentiality or the need to complete a data request form or sign a confidentiality agreement. The registrar may need to refer the requestor to the appropriate committee or IRB.

Similar issues apply to central cancer registries. Chen [3] summarized policies and procedures currently in use by some central cancer registries to respond to requests by public health officials or researchers who wish to use registry data for in-house health department programs or external research. The procedures that she provided as an example stipulate that:

- Requests for use of registry data for research must be made in writing.
- A detailed outline of the research project should be approved by an IRB.
- Provisions for protecting confidential data and preventing the unwarranted disclosure of data should be included in the application.
- There should be a written agreement that the data will be used solely for the specified research purpose.
- The data will not be released or disclosed to any unauthorized persons.
- The written request should be reviewed by a research committee for scientific merit.

As Chen [3] explained, written requests to use registry data for research purposes should be approved by an IRB. The purpose of research ethics committees or IRBs is to ensure that studies involving human research participants are designed to conform to relevant ethical standards. The requirement that research protocols undergo review by such institutional committees ensures that the rights and welfare of participants are protected and that there is a favorable balance of potential benefits and risks [17, 28]. IRBs also ensure that the proposed procedures for obtaining the informed consent of participants are adequate and that there is equity in the selection of subjects.

In the United States, federal regulations require that institutions receiving federal research funds have an interdisciplinary IRB complete a review of all research protocols [28]. The regulations provide for the expedited review or exemption of certain types of low-risk studies. Nonresearch public health practice activities such as outbreak investigations are normally exempt from IRB review.

There is also a responsibility to ensure that registry data are only used for studies with a valid design and address an important scientific question [29]. Review of research protocols should make certain that:

- The key investigators have significant training and experience in biomedical research as demonstrated by a history of prior research and publication of results in peer-reviewed journals. For student proposals, faculty committee members should posses these qualifications.
- The background reason for the proposed study is compelling as judged by the importance of the scientific question being asked, relative to fields of epidemiology, medicine, public health, or other medical research.
- The goals are clearly stated, consistent with the scientific question, and relevant to the field.
- If appropriate, sample size or power calculations indicate a reasonable chance of identifying expected differences between groups.
- The statistical techniques to be used in the data analysis, including methods to address biases in the study, are clear and appropriately used.

Maintaining Public Trust

Cancer registry professionals promote and preserve public confidence by maintaining high standards of conduct (NCRA Code of Ethics, Section I, Part A). Other measures cancer registry professionals should take to maintain public trust (and the trust of other health professionals) include communicating ethical requirements to colleagues, confronting unacceptable conduct, and avoiding conflicts of interest. For example, a conflict of interest can occur if a cancer registrar accepts compensation in return for releasing data to an outside party such as a pharmaceutical firm. The NCRA Code of Ethics [1] explain how cancer registrars should avoid conflicting interests by making "judgments and decisions without personal bias or prejudice" (Section I, Part A). Institutional policies on conflicts of interests provide additional safeguards. The NCRA Code of Ethics (Section I, Part B) also discusses the need to confront unacceptable conduct: "Do not place loyalty above duty by protecting a fellow cancer registrar who is guilty of unfair or unethical practices. Questions of conduct should be referred to the Ethics Committee for review and evaluation" [1].

Cancer registry professionals also maintain public trust by safeguarding the confidentiality and privacy of health information and by supporting registry-based studies and cancer control programs that address important health problems [1, 3]. One mechanism by which researchers who conduct registry-based studies can foster community support and trust is to establish community advisory committees to facilitate the planning, conduct, and reporting of community interventions aimed at preventing cancer or restoring health [17]. Cancer control programs that involve greater community participation and collaboration are more likely to help build public trust, to provide long-term benefits, and to develop competencies in the community.

Summary and Conclusions

The ethical precepts of cancer registration examined in this paper illustrate that many interesting and important issues vital to protecting the public's health and maintaining public trust arise in cancer registries. Cancer registrars and epidemiologists and other cancer registry professionals need to be well informed about these issues because they are central to the maintenance and utilization of cancer registry data. Additional issues that might be addressed in future ethics frameworks include the responsibilities of cancer registry professionals to communicate with community members and ethical problems arising as a result of the investigation of cancer clusters [17, 30]. For example, the identification of disease clusters in a community can lead to stigmatization of the community or its members. Ethical issues arising in registry-based cancer genetics studies also need to be further analyzed and clarified because of concern over genetic discrimination and the need to protect the privacy and confidentiality of genetic information. Another issue that might be addressed in future ethics frameworks is the need to pursue professional responsibilities diligently and to advance the cancer registry profession.

Emerging issues related to confidentiality and privacy protection, access to data, registry-based cancer genetics research, and the use of the Internet to disseminate cancer registry data require careful ethical analyses and periodically updated codes of ethics, ethics guidelines, and policy statements [3, 9, 10, 20]. Ethics codes and guidelines are not static documents, but should be periodically revisited and updated. Nevertheless, the codes and guidelines do not provide an exhaustive account of the ethical obligations of cancer registrars and those who work in central cancer registries. Specific decisions in particular cases require judgments based on the core values and ethical obligations described in the codes and guidelines and in other ethics frameworks for cancer registry professionals.

References

1. The National Cancer Registrars Association. Guide to the Interpretation of the Code of Ethics (established 1986, revised 1995). In: Hutchinson, C.L., S.D. Roffers, and A.G. Fritz, editors, *Cancer Registry Management: Principles and Practice*. Dubuque, IA: Kendall/Hunt (1997): 459–68.
2. Coleman, M.P., C.S. Muir, and F. Menegoz. Confidentiality in the Cancer Registry. *Br J Cancer* (1992):66:1138–1149.
3. Chen, V.W. The Right to Know vs. the Right to Privacy. *J Registry Manag* (1997):125:7.
4. Stiller, C.A. Cancer Registration: Its Uses in Research, and Confidentiality in the European Community. *J Epidemiol Community Health* (1993):47:342–324.
5. Muir, C.S., and E. Demaret. Cancer Registration: Legal Aspects and Confidentiality. In: Jensen, O.M., D.M. Parkin, R. MacLennan, et al., editors, *Cancer Registration: Principles and Methods*. Lyon, France: International Agency for Research on Cancer: *IARC Scientific Publications* (1991):95:199–207.
6. Bellach, B., and D. Schon. Legislation to Protect the Individual Confidentiality: the Case of Cancer Registration in Germany. *Sci Total Environ* (1996):184:33–36.

7. APHA Policy Statement 9515. *Protecting Confidential Data in Disease Registries*. Washington, D.C.: American Public Health Association (1995).

8. Watkins, S. Legal and Ethical Aspects of Cancer Data. In: Hutchinson, C.L., S.D. Roffers, and A.G. Fritz, editors, *Cancer Registry Management: Principles and Practice*. Dubuque, IA: Kendal/Hunt (1997):9–16.

9. Gostin, L.O., Z. Lazzarini, V.S. Neslund, et al. The Public Health Information Infrastructure. A National Review of the Law on Health Information Privacy. *JAMA* (1996):275:1921–1927.

10. Gold, E.B. Confidentiality and Privacy Protection in Epidemiologic Research. In: Coughlin, S.S., and T.L. Beauchamp, editors, *Ethics and Epidemiology*. New York, NY: Oxford University Press (1996):128–141.

11. Melton, L.J. Sounding Board: the Threat to Medical-Records Research. *N Engl J Med* (1997):337:1466–1469.

12. Coughlin, S.S., C.L. Soskolne, and K.W. Goodman. *Case Studies in Public Health Ethics*. Washington, D.C.: American Public Health Association (1997).

13. Overton, P., and K.J. McCracken. Using the NCRA Code of Ethics: Responsible Reporting. *The Connection* (1997):16.

14. *The Belmont Report: Ethical Principles and Guidelines for the Protection of Human Subjects of Research*. Washington, D.C.: National Commission for the Protection of Human Subjects of Biomedical and Behavioral Research (1978).

15. Beauchamp, T.L. Moral Foundations. In: Coughlin, S.S., and T.L. Beauchamp, editors, *Ethics and Epidemiology*. New York, NY: Oxford University Press (1996):24–52.

16. Clive, R.E., and D.S. Miller. Introduction to Cancer Registries: the Role of the Cancer Registrar in Cancer Control. In: Hutchinson, C.L., S.D. Roffers, and A.G. Fritz, editors, *Cancer Registry Management: Principles and Practice*. Dubuque, IA: Kendall/Hunt (1997):1–8.

17. Coughlin, S.S. Ethics in Epidemiology and Public Health Practice. In: Coughlin, S.S., editor, *Ethics in Epidemiology and Public Health Practice: Collected Works*. Columbus, GA: Quill Publications (1997):9–26.

18. Hahn, R.A. Ethical Issues. In: Teutsch, S.M., and R.E. Churchill, editors, *Principles and Practice of Public Health Surveillance*. New York, NY: Oxford University Press (1994):175–89.

19. Shultz, M.M. Legal and Ethical Considerations for Securing Consent to Epidemiologic Research in the United States. In: Coughlin, S.S., and T.L. Beauchamp, editors, *Ethics and Epidemiology*. New York, NY: Oxford University Press (1996):97–127.

20. Siwicki, B. Health Data Security: A New Priority. *Health Data Manag* (1997):5(9):46–58, 66–71.

21. Seiffert, S.E., editor. *Standards for Cancer Registries, Vol. III. Standards for Completeness, Quality, Analysis, and Management of Data*. North American Association of Central Cancer Registries (1994).

22. *Standards of the Commission on Cancer: Vol. I. Cancer Program Standards*. Chicago, IL: American College of Surgeons (1996).

23. Janes, G.R., G.C. Clutter, and M.S. Greenberg. The Health Insurance Portability and Accountability Act: New Standards for Health Data Systems. *J Registry Manag* (1998):86–90.

24. MIT Research Reveals How Public Use Data Files May Not Be Confidential After All. Assuring Privacy a Particular Challenge for Epidemiologists. *Epidemiol Monit* (1998):19:4–12.

25. Howe, H.H. Recommendations for Public Use Files of National Cancer Data. A report of a workshop held at the Broadmoor, Colorado Springs, CO, August 25–27, 1997. North American Association of Central Cancer Registries (1997).

26. Coughlin, S.S. Ethically Optimized Study Designs in Epidemiology. In: Coughlin, S.S., and T.L. Beauchamp, editors, *Ethics and Epidemiology*. New York, NY: Oxford University Press (1996):145–155.

27. *Standards of the Commission on Cancer, Vol. 2: Registry Operations and Data Standards.* Chicago, IL: American College of Surgeons (1997).
28. Levine, R.J. The Institutional Review Board. In: Coughlin, S.S., and T.L. Beauchamp, editors, *Ethics and Epidemiology.* New York, NY: Oxford University Press (1996):257–273.
29. Title 25. Health Services. Part I. Texas Department of Health. Chapter 37. Maternal and Child Health Services. Surveillance and Control of Birth Defects. 25 TAC 37.301–37.306. Texas Register October 7, 1994: 8032-6.
30. Guidelines for Investigating Clusters of Health Events. *MMWR* (1990):39(RR-11):1–16.

CHAPTER 7

ORGANIZATIONAL ETHICS AND PUBLIC HEALTH PRACTICE

S.S. Coughlin, D.H. Barrett, and R.E. Dixon

Members of the public and stakeholder groups depend on public health agencies to safeguard the health and safety of their families and communities. Public health officials are accountable both to the public and to elected officials and governing bodies with oversight responsibilities [1]. Moreover, United States Federal agencies such as the Centers for Disease Control and Prevention (CDC), which employ many professional epidemiologists, scientists, administrators, and other professionals recognized as experts in their field, enjoy well-deserved international reputations for excellence in public health research and practice. Similarly, academic institutions, including schools of public health and medicine, also employ many outstanding public health scientists who are accountable to their employer, students, their profession, funding agencies, and the public.

Public health professionals, health advocates, elected officials, and other persons with vested interests in the integrity, well-being, and continued progress of the public health enterprise have witnessed a range of ethical dilemmas and issues involving public health agencies and biomedical institutions. These ethical concerns, including some cases brought to public attention by whistle-blowers, have involved federal, state, or local health agencies as well as major universities. Focus groups have suggested that ethical issues encountered by public health practitioners in the United States relate to public–private partnerships and collaborations, the allocation of scarce resources, setting of priorities, and choosing among different groups and health needs, the collection and use of data and information, and politics and relationships with other government officials and legislative bodies [2]. Surveys of public health practitioners demonstrate that ethical issues such as conflicts of interest and political pressure occur at the state and local levels [1, 2]. Other reported ethical problems included reports of conflicts of interest, instances of inadvertent release of confidential medical information by leading government agencies and health care organizations and institutions, and charges by government scientists that their research findings had been delayed or altered. These controversies occur at the intersection of politics and public health, partly because of the importance of these public health and biomedical research institutions to the public good. Alleged instances of conflicts of interest, retaliation against whistle-blowers, and other ethical problems can also be viewed in the context of public health ethics, organizational ethics, and professional ethics.

Despite the enormity and breadth of these challenges, the sizable literature on ethical issues in epidemiology and public health practice has paid surprisingly little attention to organizational ethics. Even when authors have examined ethics at public health institutions, they have rarely considered the linkages between organizational ethics, professional ethics, or ethics frameworks for dealing with tensions and challenges inherent in public health. For example, the National Working Group on Health Care Organizational Ethics convened by the Institute of Ethics at the American Medical Association, focused on organizations that provide health care to individual patients, but did not address organizational ethics at federal or state government agencies [3]. In addition, seminal articles on public health ethics have tended to compare and contrast public health ethics with medical ethics rather than delve deeply into organizational ethics concepts or frameworks. In this article, we summarize current concepts of organizational ethics, and identify frameworks, guidelines, and procedures that are likely to be helpful in improving and sustaining ethics at public health institutions and organizations. This discussion includes a summary of stakeholder theory and accountability in public health. To provide a case study, we summarize the activities of the CDC Public Health Ethics Committee (PHEC). A consideration of these topics supports the conclusion that public health professionals and oversight bodies should devote greater attention to organizational ethics and professional ethics at public health institutions.

Organizational Ethics

The ethics of an organization is intertwined with an organization's culture and partly relates to how it responds to an internal or external stimulus or prompt (e.g., reports of a public health threat or concern that is not adequately being addressed). As noted by Ells and MacDonald [4], "organizational ethics is the study and practice of the ethical behavior of organizations. It involves clarifying and evaluating the values embedded in organizational policies and practices and seeking mechanisms for establishing morally acceptable values-based practices and policies." Organizational ethics expresses the values of an organization to its employees and stakeholders. Values contribute to the culture and ultimate success of organizations [5]. Whether they are nonprofit or for-profit, private or public, ethical organizations are likely to have enhanced abilities to recruit and retain experienced and knowledgeable employees [6]. In the discussion that follows, several organizational ethics strategies are noted that seek to prevent ethical problems rather than react to ethical problems as they arise [4]. Organizational ethics can be seen as a set of tools that can be used for fostering accountability and improving the ethical climate of an organization.

Elements of Organizational Ethics

Key elements of an organization's ethics include a written code of ethics and institutional ethics policies and standards, ongoing ethics training for all employees including executives and managers, the availability of ethics consultation, and ongoing systems for the reporting of ethical problems and concerns. Examples of codes of ethics include those drafted by the Public Health Leadership Society and the American College of Health Care Administrators [7, 8]. In public health practice and management, organizational ethics "involves providing public health leaders and workers with training, tools, and organizational structures, such as committees, to help them recognize the ethical dimensions of their work and integrate the agency's values into the performance of their tasks" [9]. At the CDC, for example, the focus of the PHEC is on improving public health practice rather than compliance or risk management [10]. Public health ethics activities at the agency, including continuing education on public health ethics and procedures for ethics consultation, are part of a larger group of ethics-related activities such as those pertaining to the maintenance and enforcement of scientific integrity, addressing conflicts of interest or other employee conduct issues, regulatory activities, and protecting human subjects in research [10]. Institutional ethics committees help to overcome what Boyle and colleagues [11] referred to as "moral silence," that is, the failure of some employees or organizations to articulate and act on their moral convictions. They may also counter the perception that considering the ethical implications of organizational practices is naïve, idealistic, inefficient, or impractical [11].

Protection of Whistle-Blowers

In order for consultation and reporting systems to be successful, an environment must exist in which there is zero tolerance for retaliation against persons seeking to report ethics problems or to receive consultation about an ethical concern. Whistle-blowing is often an effort by a member of an organization to convey information to person(s) inside or outside the organization concerning a serious wrongdoing or danger created or masked by the organization [12]. Information may be revealed about illegal, inefficient, or wasteful activities that endanger the health, safety, or freedom of the public [13]. Darr [13] argued that blowing the whistle inside of an organization is more likely to be viewed as positive because the organization has an opportunity to correct the problem. However, employees may face adverse repercussions from both internal and external whistle-blowing despite the No Fear Act and other legal protections. Conflicts in values inherent to whistle-blowing often include a tension between loyalty to clients or personal values versus loyalty to the organization [12, 14]. Whistle-blower protection laws and institutional policies go hand in hand with measures to bolster organizational ethics such as the formation of ethics committees and ethics consultation procedures, the provision of ethics education, the adoption of codes of ethics, and linkages of ethics activities with measures for quality control and accountability. Conflict resolution training for all employees is also likely to be helpful.

Leadership Theories and Organizational Ethics

The importance of organizational values has been extensively discussed in the literature on management and leadership [5]. Studies have shown that successful leaders frequently have inspiring values. In addition, leadership writers and theorists have increasingly described values, principles, or ethics as key components of effective leadership and as essential traits for leaders [5]. Numerous theories and frameworks for organizational ethics have been proposed, reflecting the diversity of theories of management, leadership, human resources, psychology, and business ethics.

The framework of transformational leadership, which focuses on synergistic change, was articulated by James Burns [15] in the 1970s. In Burns' view, leadership involves the clarification of values and the uncovering of contradictions among values and between values and practice, and the realigning of values with the needs of the organization. Subsequent authors, including Stephen Covey [16], have argued that our values should be aligned with certain principles, in order to provide effective leadership (hence the terms "principle-based" or "values-based leadership"). Covey [16] suggested that the goal of a transformational leader is "to transform people and organizations in a literal sense, to change them in mind and heart; enlarge vision, insight and understanding; clarify purposes; make behavior congruent with beliefs, principles, or values; and bring about changes that are permanent, self perpetuating, and momentum-building." Charismatic and servant leadership theories also have potential relevance to organizational ethics [17]. Whereas (secular) charismatic leaders strive to reframe followers' perceptions of the nature of their work, to frame an appealing future vision, and to develop a collective identity among employees, servant leaders see leadership as an opportunity to help others to achieve their full potential, to practice authenticity, and to build community [17–19]. In any organization, organizational ethics are strongly influenced by leadership, partly because leaders help to shape the organization's vision, goals, objectives, strategic plans, and values. Nevertheless, it is desirable for communication, discussion, and debate about ethics and values to occur throughout all areas of an organization, from small teams to much larger groups, so that organizational members are empowered to help implement and shape the organization's values and goals. Examples of commonly cited values include truth (veracity), trust, mentoring, openness (transparency), giving credit, and caring. For many writers on organizational ethics, leaders are not the sole or primary source of an organization's values. Rather, shared principles, values, and mission statements are developed using a participative process [5].

In business ethics models, organizational ethics relates to corporate governance and corporate ethics [6]. Business ethics is generally concerned with the decision-making of organizations and managers, including the fiduciary obligations of managers and organizations to stockholders and responsibilities to other stakeholders. Although the literature on business ethics and corporate leadership deals with many topics of potential interest to public health leaders, ethical considerations in preventive health care and public health—including organizational ethics at government public health agencies—are unlikely to be satisfactorily addressed by directly applying accounts of ethics derived from the for-profit business sector. Scholars have argued that health care in the United States is viewed as a special type of good that cannot be dealt with ethically in the same fashion as most other commodities in the marketplace. Nevertheless, some concepts discussed and debated in the literature on business ethics and management (e.g., stakeholder models and theory) are of potential interest to considerations of organizational ethics in public health practice.

Stakeholder Models and Stakeholder Theory

Stakeholders consist of individuals or groups whose role relationships with an organization help to define the organization, its mission, purpose, or goals, and are affected by the organization's activities [20, 21]. For example, public health professionals have role obligations to their employer, their profession, funders, and the communities they serve. In addition to describing stakeholder relationships internally and externally, an organization's stakeholders can also be prioritized in terms of their importance or influence. Because an organization and its stakeholders can affect the other in terms of harms (e.g., adversely affecting its well-being) and benefits (e.g., helping to ensure the success of an organization), stakeholder relationships can be viewed as "normative reciprocal relationships for which each party is accountable" [21]. The adequacy of relationships with stakeholders can be judged according to principles of fairness (e.g., using the approach advocated by Rawls [22]), respect for persons, procedural justice, or other formal criteria or standards.

Stakeholder theory, which has frequently been cited in the literature on business ethics, has potentially useful applications to organizational ethics in health care and public health, especially where there is a need to describe, prescribe, or derive alternatives for organizational leadership that balance a multitude of interests [21, 23]. As Werhane [21] put it, "stakeholder theory initiates thinking about organization ethics . . . while including the stakeholder dimensions of professional, clinical, and managerial ethics." Although stakeholder theory was initially proposed in the context of the strategic management of private sector firms [21], more recent authors have applied it to managerial decision-making in the public sector including government agencies. Stakeholder theories sometimes assume that an organization and all its stakeholders form a shared moral community. In some formulations, stakeholder theory appeals to principles of fairness when evaluating organizational decisions. Various approaches to stakeholder analysis have been proposed including normative, instrumental, and descriptive [4, 24]. For example, the manner in which an organization's employees or managers actually behave may be analyzed and described. A second approach—normative—considers the manner in which managers and employees should behave. This approach goes beyond simply describing stakeholder relationships to recommend certain organizational structures and practices and managerial attitudes that, taken as a whole, constitute stakeholder management [24]. As a third approach, certain outcomes may be determined to be more likely if employees or managers behave in certain ways; this instrumental approach holds that the practice of stakeholder management is related to various performance goals of the organization.

Although courses and lectures on management attended by public health professionals sometimes include a diagram representing a "stakeholder model" or other descriptions of stakeholders, it is important to consider why one stakeholder theory or model should be preferred over any alternative conception [24]. Particular conceptions of stakeholder theories and models have not been adequately addressed in the context of public health practice or research. In addition, concepts of stakeholder model, stakeholder management, and stakeholder theory have been explained differently by various authors and supported with diverse and sometimes inconsistent arguments [24]. Further work is needed to fully evaluate applications of stakeholder theory to public health and biomedical research organizations and agencies. For example, an instrumental justification of a particular stakeholder theory should identify connections between the theory and organizational performance. Normative justifications should appeal to underlying moral concepts such as utilitarianism, individual or group rights, or fairness [24]. Stakeholder theory may facilitate the prioritization of those affecting and affected by the organization and clarify the reciprocal accountability relationships that have been described in the literature on professional ethics, medicine, and public health (e.g., the obligations that health professionals have toward patients and community members), but which have not always been connected to organizational accountability [21].

Accountability

Accountability involves the procedures and processes by which one individual or organization justifies and takes responsibility for its activities [25]. As previously noted, public health agencies are accountable to the public and to oversight bodies. Baum and colleagues [26] observed that the responsible and competent stewardship of public funds contributes to accountability. In addition to financial responsibility and performance, accountability has several domains with relevance to public health agencies. These include professional competence, legal and ethical conduct, adequacy of access to public health services, public health promotion, and community benefit [25]. Transparency (i.e., making public and explicit one's assumptions, justifications, and reasoning) also contributes to the accountability of public health agencies, since transparency is essential for establishing trust with the public [26].

The responsibility for moral actions can be viewed as ultimately resting with individuals rather than organizational systems or processes [27]. As Potter [27] put it, individuals should speak out of "conviction as to what is right and just" and display virtues such as courage and persistence in standing up for what is right and helping to mobilize an appropriate response when ethical concerns arise. Nevertheless, several authors have argued that health care organizations are ethically accountable for their actions, especially if identifiable decision-making processes exist and there is sufficient coordination among the efforts of individual persons within the organization. Emanuel [28], for example, argued that moral demands exist not only on the individual but also on organizations, systems, and institutions. Within any organization, managerial and administrative individuals are frequently designated with the function of taking on the organization's responsibility. Thus, it is reasonable to conclude that organizations are moral agents that can be held morally accountable, even though they are not moral agents in the same sense as individuals [21].

The Intersection of Organizational Ethics and Professional Ethics

In contrast to organizational ethics and public health ethics, the domains of professional ethics include ethical duties and obligations within individual professions such as medicine or epidemiology. Within each profession, widely shared ethical norms have often been codified as professional codes of conduct or ethics guidelines. Examples include ethics guidelines developed for epidemiologists and other public health professionals. Frameworks for professional ethics often take into account the distinctive history and tradition of a given profession as well as special obligations and permissions granted to that profession by society in accordance with particular professional roles (e.g., the responsibilities and authority that medical doctors bear to care for patients who are sick or injured). As noted elsewhere in this volume, public health ethics, which has different domains from those of medical ethics, organizational ethics, or professional ethics, can be defined as the identification, analysis, and resolution of ethical problems arising in public health practice and research.

Previous authors have provided accounts of ethics activities pursued by professional associations within such fields as epidemiology and health services management [11, 29, 30]. Bernheim and Melnick [9] provided an account of organizational ethics and professional ethics in public health practice and management. They noted that "Leadership requires an ongoing approach to ethics that focuses on two dimensions of practice: the professional relationships of officials developed over time with their communities and the ethical aspects of day-to-day public health activities" [9]. Public health professionals may build and sustain positive relationships with community members, and seek public input about challenging ethical issues, through consultation with community representatives and advisory committees. Measures such as public engagement, focus groups involving members of the general public, and seeking public comment from stakeholder groups and community members may nurture civic cooperation and trust in public health agencies [9].

In public health practice and management, conflicts in values can occur due to conflicting values across professional groups or institutions. For example, there may be a conflict between achieving quality and reducing costs, or between serving an individual or the community. The inclusion of numerous professional and nonprofessional groups within public health agencies adds to the heterogeneity of value systems and cultures within public health organizations. Ambiguous or conflicting values (e.g., a system that rewards behaviors that are inconsistent with accountability and protecting the public's health through effective and efficient science-based programs, or professional ethics) can lead to uncertainty about what the organization really wants to achieve and decrease employee motivation or morale. As Graber and Kilpatrick [5] put it, "It is clearly not enough to profess important values only at the top of the organization or in written statements of core values. Those at the top must establish mechanisms that reward those who enact these values." In situations where value systems are noted to be incongruous, public health professionals should ideally work with other like-minded professionals to change the organizational culture so that it has "strong values that organizational members can embrace and adhere to" [5].

A further issue is that many organizational ethics issues also have legal implications, that is, there is overlap with public health law. Government employees are subject to a variety of Federal laws, regulations, and policies that seek to prevent moral problems such as discrimination in hiring and promotion, and retaliation against whistle-blowers (e.g., the No Fear Act). Conflicts related to employee hiring, promotion, and termination can be related both to Federal law, regulations, and institutional policies and to organizational ethics [9]. Although ethical and legal requirements are often seamless, attempts to combine Federal laws and regulations, public health ethics, professional ethics, and business ethics do not always result in identical guides for decision-making or action.

Organizational Ethics and Public Health Ethics

Overlap exists between organizational ethics and other areas of applied ethics including public health ethics, medical ethics, professional ethics, and government ethics. As noted elsewhere in this volume, public health ethics can be defined as the identification, analysis, and resolution of ethical problems arising in public health practice and research. Childress et al. [31] noted that public health ethics includes a loose set of general moral considerations (values, principles, or rules) that are relevant to public health. Accounts of public health ethics commonly point to principles such as beneficence and justice and important rules and values such as ensuring public participation and the participation of affected parties (procedural justice), protecting privacy and confidentiality, keeping promises and commitments, speaking honestly and disclosing information (transparency), and building and maintaining public trust. Other important values for the practice of public health are effectiveness, efficiency, proportionality, necessity, least infringement, and public justification. Public health ethics has different domains from those of medical ethics, organizational ethics, or professional ethics. To illustrate how the domains of organizational ethics and public health ethics intersect and complement each other, we provide the following case study of the activities of the CDC PHEC.

CDC Public Health Ethics Activities

The CDC, the nation's premier public health agency, is charged with promoting health and improving quality of life by preventing and controlling disease, injury, and disability. CDC accomplishes its mission by working within the United States and, by invitation from foreign governments and professional colleagues, throughout the world to monitor health, detect and investigate health problems, conduct research to enhance prevention, develop and advocate for sound public health policies, implement prevention strategies, promote healthy behaviors, foster safe and healthful environments, and provide leadership and training. CDC's leadership is dedicated to scientific excellence and high-quality, ethical public health practice. CDC's core values—respect, integrity, and accountability—serve as the foundation for all activities at the agency.

Ethics activities at CDC have taken a variety of forms. There are programs and policies related to maintaining and enforcing scientific integrity, addressing conflicts of interest or other employee conduct issues, and protecting human subjects in research. These are long-standing programs that fit into what has traditionally been considered the domain of organizational ethics. A more recent initiative at CDC has been its focus on public health ethics. These activities have centered on developing the capacity of CDC staff to engage in a systematic, deliberate ethical analysis of public health decisions and on the development of ethics guidance for a number of specific programmatic issues.

The need to strengthen CDC's ability to address ethical issues in the practice of public health became evident during the 2004 seasonal influenza vaccine shortage when decisions needed to be made regarding how to distribute the reduced supply of the vaccine. Additionally, planning for pandemic influenza and other public health emergencies has brought to the forefront a number of ethical issues (e.g., use of interventions that limit individual liberties, such as quarantine, and the need to prioritize who will receive vaccines, antiviral medications, and other resources that may be in limited supply).

CDC's public health ethics activities illustrate how organizational ethics and public health ethics complement each other. Public health ethics can help in public health decision-making by building and maintaining credibility and public trust in agency decisions, by fostering consensus and resolving values conflicts in an atmosphere of respect for stakeholders, and by assisting in decision-making when there is scientific uncertainty and many perspectives about how to proceed. Although ethical decision-making has always been integral to all CDC decision-making, a systematic, deliberate ethical analysis provides added value by ensuring that public health decision-making is consistent with public health values and that decisions are supported by those affected by public health actions.

Public health ethics is not about finding fault or assigning blame. It is principally about improving public health practice, particularly public health decision-making at the program level. The application of public health ethics differs from CDC's other ethics-related activities because it is not oriented toward enforcement or assuring compliance with regulations, guidelines, or standards of employee behavior. The primary purpose of applying public health ethics is to help inform decision-makers, whether managers or program staff, so that they can better address and resolve ethical dilemmas in public health. The expectation is that integrating a systematic ethical analysis for public health decision-making at CDC will result in benefits such as increased transparency in decision-making, enhanced public trust, strengthened scientific integrity, and increased capacity of CDC staff to recognize and address ethical issues.

CDC Public Health Ethics infrastructure. In early 2005, CDC launched its initiative to strengthen leadership in public health ethics. The main elements of this initiative are the Ethics Subcommittee of the Advisory Committee to the Director (Ethics Subcommittee, ACD) and the CDC PHEC. The Ethics Subcommittee, ACD was established to provide counsel to CDC on a broad range of public health ethics questions and issues arising from programs, scientists, and practitioners, and to support CDC in the development of the internal capacity to identify, analyze, and resolve ethical issues. The Ethics Subcommittee, ACD is composed of academic and professional ethicists from outside CDC who serve up to 4 years. The Ethics Subcommittee of the ACD has worked with CDC on developing a number of ethics guidance documents. These include guidance for public health emergency preparedness and response, for addressing pandemic influenza planning and response, and for use of travel restrictions for the control of infectious diseases.

The mission of the internal CDC committee, PHEC, is to provide leadership in public health ethics at CDC and to work with CDC staff to integrate the tools of ethical analysis into decisions and day-to-day activities across CDC. PHEC is composed of representatives from each of CDC's national centers and from other organizational components within CDC (e.g., offices within the Office of the Director, Coordinating Center offices, and science-related workgroups). Although there are no specific criteria for membership on PHEC other than an interest in public health ethics and a commitment to strengthening CDC's ability to systematically apply ethical principles to public health decision-making, PHEC members are expected to participate in ongoing training sponsored by the committee.

Two important components of PHEC's activities are to provide education to PHEC members and other CDC staff on public health ethics and to develop the capacity to conduct public health ethics consultations. The PHEC Education Subcommittee is responsible for assessing CDC resources, needs, and competency relating to public health ethics; for planning educational programs in public health ethics for CDC staff; for conducting competency-based trainings, workshops, seminars; and for evaluating public health ethics educational and training activities. The PHEC Consult Subcommittee takes the lead on public health ethics consultations using a systematic approach to clarifying the issue, determining the pertinent ethical principles and values, identifying possible alternative courses of action and ethical arguments for and against each proposed action, recommending a strategy, and evaluating the outcome.

An example of CDC's public health ethics activities is the guidance released in March 2007 that provides a general ethical framework for decision-making relating to pandemic influenza planning and response. "Ethical Guidelines in Pandemic Influenza" includes a discussion of general ethical considerations as well as specific ethical considerations relating to vaccine and antiviral drug distribution and the development of interventions that would limit individual freedoms for the protection of the public good [32]. This document serves as a resource for CDC decision-makers as well as CDC's state and local partners for the development of pandemic influenza control plans.

Additional observations. CDC's commitment to strengthening the capacity of its staff to systematically identify, clarify, analyze, and resolve ethical issues that inevitably develop in the day-to-day decision-making and actions relating to the protection of the public's health illustrate how a focus on public health ethics can complement the other ethics activities conducted by the agency. A focus on public health ethics has strengthened CDC organizational ethics by clarifying and emphasizing its commitments to transparency and openness in decision-making, to sharing information with and obtaining input from the public, to making decisions based on the best available scientific information. It also provides a formal mechanism for CDC staff to safely raise concerns about the agency's practices and decisions.

It is anticipated that as the public health ethics activities grow within CDC's organizational components, benefits will be seen in greater participation and partnership with affected stakeholders and strengthened public trust in health recommendations. As the nation moves forward to address traditional public health issues as well as other complex health threats, such as pandemic illnesses and large-scale man-made and natural emergency events, health decisions must be based on a clear ethical foundation that serves as a guide to public health decision-making.

Summary and Conclusions

Organizations, systems, and institutions in health care and public health are composed of individuals and groups of people with moral obligations [28]. Although this essay has considered several important topics related to organizational ethics and public health, more scholarly work in this area is needed. For example, issues for which individual public health professionals and organizations are to be accountable are only partly identified in existing practice guidelines, ethics guidelines, and codes of conduct. In addition, recommendations from existing codes and guidelines are sometimes nonspecific and open to alternative interpretations, or lack mechanisms of enforcement to ensure compliance and accountability. In practice, the accountability of public health institutions often exists at a relatively high and abstract level.

The common understanding of an organization's mission, vision, and values is an important underpinning to organizational ethics. A strong, ethical culture with shared values is likely to enhance organizational performance by maximizing motivation among staff. As Darr [13] put it, "shared values and behaviors make staff feel good about working for an organization." However, decisions made by public health leaders or managers must be consistent with organizational values or employees may conclude that leaders are being inconsistent or hypocritical.

A further issue is that experts may disagree about the scope of organizational ethics or about the relationship of organizational ethics to other areas of ethics. Organizational ethics at public health agencies and institutions is likely to overlap with public health ethics and other areas of applied ethics (e.g., professional ethics in such fields as epidemiology, medicine, emergency response, and government service). Nevertheless, frameworks for organizational ethics—which extend beyond public health to include many other areas of government and the private sector including nonprofit and for-profit organizations and institutions—are likely to include useful tools for addressing ethical issues at public health agencies and institutions. Organizational ethics frameworks explicitly take into account the level of analysis or moral vantage point (e.g., analyses that occur at the level of individuals, teams, institutions, or health systems, including interactions between various levels of analysis). This does not mean that organizational ethics frameworks should replace those based on public health ethics. Rather, the two are likely to be complementary. As one sign of the usefulness of organizational ethics, the Joint Commission on Accreditation of Health Care Organizations requires health care organizations such as hospitals, nursing homes, home care agencies, hospices, and integrated delivery systems to identify and address organizational ethics [11].

When an ethical problem or dilemma is encountered within a public health institution, public health values such as transparency, openness of communication, and protecting the public welfare should be paramount. However, public health values may sometimes be seen to be in conflict with other values that are frequently cited in government and business, such as those pertaining to the tension between scientific or academic freedom versus the desirability of agencies speaking with one voice, and the need to balance transparency with privacy concerns. In such situations of values conflicts, institutional resources for ethics consultation, systems for the reporting of ethical problems and concerns, and monitoring and evaluation may be especially helpful [33]. In order for consultation and reporting systems to be successful, persons reporting ethical problems must be protected from retaliation in accordance with whistle-blower protection laws and institutional policies. Efforts to strengthen organizational ethics, such as programs for ethics consultation, ethics education, government or academic ethics compliance, institutional structures to strengthen accountability, and opportunities to express disagreement within the organization, are likely to minimize the perceived necessity of whistle-blowing and foster public trust in public health agencies and institutions.

Acknowledgments

The findings and conclusions in this article are those of the authors and do not necessarily represent the official position of the CDC or Department of Veterans Affairs.

References

1. Gollust, S.E., N.M. Baum, and P.D. Jacobson. Politics and Public Health Ethics in Practice: Right and Left Meet Right and Wrong. *J Public Health Manag Pract* (2008):14:340–347.
2. Bernheim, R.G. Public Health Ethics: The Voices of Practitioners. *J Law Med Ethics* (2003):31 (4 Suppl):104–109.
3. Ozar, D., J. Berg, P.H. Werhane, and L. Emanuel. *Organizational Ethics in Healthcare. Toward a Model for Ethical Decision-Making by Provider Organizations.* Institute for Ethics National Working Group. Chicago, IL: American Medical Association (1999).
4. Ells, C., and C. MacDonald. Implications of Organizational Ethics to Healthcare. *Healthc Manage Forum* (2002):15:32–38.
5. Graber, D.R., and A.O. Kilpatrick. Establishing Values-Based Leadership and Value Systems in Healthcare Organizations. *J Health Hum Serv Adm* (2008):31:179–197.
6. Driscoll, D.M., and W.M. Howffman. *Ethics Matters: How to Implement Values-Driven Management.* Waltham, MA: Bently College Center for Business Ethics (2000).
7. Public Health Leadership Society. *Principles of the Ethical Practice of Public Health* (2002). Available at http://www.apha.org/NR/rdonlyres/1CED3CEA-287E-4185-9CBD-BD405FC60856/0/ethicsbrochure.pdf. Accessed April 6, 2009.
8. American College of Healthcare Executives (ACHE) Code of Ethics. In: Darr, K., editor, *Ethics in Health Services Management* (4th ed.). Baltimore, MD: Health Professions Press (2005):361–364.
9. Bernheim, R.G., and A. Melnick. Principled Leadership in Public Health: Integrating Ethics into Practice and Management. *J Public Health Manag Pract* (2008):14:358–366.
10. Barrett, D.H., R.H. Bernier, and A.L. Sowell. Strengthening Public Health Ethics at the Centers for Disease Control and Prevention. *J Public Health Manag Pract* (2008):14:348–353.

11. Boyle, P.J., E.R. DuBose, S.J. Ellingson, et al. *Organizational Ethics in Health Care. Principles, Cases, and Practical Solutions*. San Francisco, CA: Jossey-Bass (2001).

12. Lachman, V.D. Whistleblowing: Role of Organizational Culture in Prevention and Management. *Medsurg Nursing* (2008):17:265–267.

13. Darr, K. *Ethics in Health Services Management* (4th ed.). Baltimore, MD: Health Professions Press (2005).

14. Ray, S.L. Whistleblowing and Organizational Ethics. *Nursing Ethics* (2006):13:438–445.

15. Burns, J.M. *Leadership*. New York, NY: Harper and Row (1978).

16. Covey, S. *Principle-Centered Leadership*. New York, NY: Free Press (1991).

17. Shamir, B., and J.M. Howell. Organizational and Contextual Influences on the Emergence and Effectiveness of Charismatic Leadership. *Leadersh Q* (1999):10:257–283.

18. Smith, B.N., R.V. Montagno, and T.N. Kuzmenko. Transformational and Servant Leadership: Content and Contextual Comparisons. *J Leadersh Organ Studies* (2004):10:80–91.

19. Caldwell, C., C. Voelker, R.D. Dixon, and A. LeJuene. Transformative Leadership: An Ethical Stewardship Model for Healthcare. *Organ Ethics* (2007):4:126–134.

20. Freeman, R.E. Strategic Management: A Stakeholder Approach. Boston, MA: Pitman (1984).

21. Werhane, P.H. Business Ethics, Stakeholder Theory, and the Ethics of Healthcare Organizations. *Camb Q Healthc Ethics* (2000):9:169–181.

22. Rawls, J. *A Theory of Justice*. Cambridge, MA: Harvard University Press (1971).

23. Jones, T.M., and A.C. Wicks. Convergent Stakeholder Theory. *Acad Manage Rev* (1999): 24:206–221.

24. Donaldson, T., and L.E. Preston. The Stakeholder Theory of the Corporation: Concepts, Evidence, and Implications. *Acad Manage Rev* (1995):20:65–91.

25. Emanuel, E.J., and L.L. Emanuel. What Is Accountability in Health Care? *Ann Intern Med* (1996):124:229–239.

26. Baum, N.M., S.E. Gollust, S.D. Goold, and P.D. Jacobson. Looking Ahead: Addressing Ethical Challenges in Public Health Practice. *J Law Med Ethics* (2007):35(4):657–667.

27. Potter, V.R. Individuals Bear Responsibility. *Bioethics Forum* (1996):12(2):27–28.

28. Emanuel, L.L. Ethics and the Structures of Healthcare. *Camb Q Healthc Ethics* (2000):9: 151–168.

29. Coughlin, S.S. On the Role of Ethics Committees in Epidemiology Professional Societies. *Am J Epidemiol* (1997):146:209–213.

30. Soskolne, C.L., and L.E. Sieswerda. Implementing Ethics in the Professions: Examples from Environmental Epidemiology. *Sci Eng Ethics* (2003):9:181–190.

31. Childress, J.F., R.R. Faden, R.D. Gaare, et al. Public Health Ethics: Mapping the Terrain. *J Law Med Ethics* (2002):30:170–178.

32. Centers for Disease Control and Prevention. *Ethical Guidelines in Pandemic Influenza* Available at http://www.cdc.gov/od/science/phethics/panFlu_Ethic_Guidelines.pdf Accessed April 6, 2009.

33. Yuspeh, A., K. Whalen, and J. Cecelic, et al. Above Reproach: Developing a Comprehensive Ethics and Compliance Program. *Front Health Serv Manage* (1999):16:3–38.

PART IV

ETHICS INSTRUCTION IN EPIDEMIOLOGY AND PUBLIC HEALTH

The readings in this section, including an article on "Model Curricula in Public Health Ethics," provide a rationale for instruction in public health ethics and attempt to foster institutional support for such efforts. Although surveys indicate that many schools of public health are offering such courses, at least on an elective basis, several graduate programs in public health do not offer or require such instruction. Part of the problem may be a shortage of trained instructors who are knowledgeable about public health ethics. However, formal instruction in public health ethics and on scientific integrity in epidemiology has burgeoned since the publication of the first edition of this book.

The Association of Schools of Public Health (ASPH) ethics survey included in this section is one of several surveys that have examined ethics instruction at public health institutions. Kessel conducted a survey of the nature and content of teaching of public health ethics in medical schools and public health graduate programs in the United Kingdom. Public health ethics was taught in 75% of medical schools and 52% of institutions providing postgraduate education, although the content and nature of ethics teaching was incomplete and often minimal [1]. In September of 2006, Agee and Gimbel assessed the availability of required and elective courses in law and ethics at accredited public health schools and programs [2]. Of the 93 programs and schools reviewed, 14% required a course in ethics. Additional ethics surveys have been conducted at U.S. institutions that train graduate students in epidemiology and other public health disciplines.

General courses on scientific integrity are required at institutions receiving funding from the National Institutes of Health (NIH). At the Centers for Disease Control and Prevention (CDC), lectures on ethics are provided to epidemiology intelligence service officers and to other CDC staff, and computerized instruction on ethics has been developed for CDC personnel. Another notable development in the past decade has been the completion of the ASPH model curricula in public health ethics. Innovative courses on ethics and epidemiology and public health ethics have been offered at several schools of public health and in graduate summer programs.

Topics dealt with in courses on ethical issues in epidemiology and public health research include a framework for ethics in health research, basic methods of moral reasoning, ethics guidelines for epidemiologists, privacy and confidentiality protection, issues surrounding informed consent, ethical issues in studies of vulnerable populations, human subjects research, communication responsibilities of epidemiologists, issues surrounding the publication of research findings, conflicts of interest, and scientific misconduct. In courses on public health ethics, students may be challenged with questions related to the ethics of priority setting for prevention and intervention. For example, who should set priorities for prevention and what criteria and measures of impact should they use? Is it a problem that funding for prevention and intervention activities is sometimes out of step with the findings of epidemiologic studies that point to certain proximal or distal risk factors for illness or injury or other social problems? Topics dealt with in the ASPH model curricula on public health ethics include the legacy of the Tuskegee Syphilis Study, human rights, public health research and practice in international settings, community-based practice and research, the ethics of infectious disease control (sexually transmitted diseases, human immunodeficiency virus, and tuberculosis), ethical issues in environmental and occupational health, public health genetics, and health system reform including access, priority setting, and allocation of resources. Priority setting and allocation of scarce resources are among the topics discussed in the recent literature on ethical issues in emergency preparedness and response (e.g., those arising in a possible pandemic of avian influenza).

1. Kessel, A.S. Public Health Ethics: Teaching Survey and Critical Review. *Soc Sci Med* (2003):56:1439–1445.
2. Agee, B., and R.W. Gimbel. Assessing the Legal and Ethical Preparedness of Master of Public Health Graduates. *Am J Public Health* (2009):99:1505–9.

CHAPTER 8

MODEL CURRICULA IN PUBLIC HEALTH ETHICS

Steven S. Coughlin

T he provision of ethics instruction through formal courses and other avenues is a cornerstone of professional ethics in public health. Key developments include the implementation of innovative ethics curricula in public health training programs in the United States and other countries, numerous ethics workshops and symposia at national and international public health meetings, and increasing opportunities for public health professionals to obtain continuing education on ethics [1–4]. Another recent development has been the NIH mandate for extramural research training programs to provide instruction on scientific integrity and ethical principles in research to trainees [5, 6].

Despite the recent upsurge of interest in the inclusion of ethics instruction in public health curricula, schools of public health and other institutions that train public health professionals vary greatly in the depth of their attention to ethics. Moreover, existing ethics curricula in public health vary considerably in their form and content, even within individual disciplines such as epidemiology [2, 4, 7]. Although innovation and creativity in teaching methods are desirable, there are currently no national standards for adequate instruction in public health ethics.

The thesis of this article is that schools of public health should provide basic instruction in ethics that is specifically tailored to meet the needs of public health students, and that model curricula in public health ethics are needed to assure this goal. Such curricula should have clearly specified and evaluable learning objectives and should take into account the diversity of public health students, disciplines, and graduate education programs. In the discussion that follows, a rationale for teaching public health ethics is provided along with some responses to possible questions.

Rationale for Teaching Public Health Ethics

In recent decades, training in medical ethics has become standard in medical and nursing education in the United States and many other countries [7–9]. Many medical specialty boards have also formally endorsed ethics teaching and evaluation for residents. Courses and seminar series on medical ethics are offered at virtually all academic medical centers in the United States [7, 9]. The basic curricular goals in medical ethics include dilemmas that arise in clinical medicine such as how to proceed if a patient refuses treatment, knowledge of the moral aspects of the care of patients with a poor prognosis, and deciding when it is morally justified to breach confidentiality [7].

"Model Curricula in Public Health Ethics" originally appeared in the American Journal of Preventive Medicine (1996):12:247–251. Used with permission of Oxford University Press.

Bioethics curricula developed for physicians-in-training do not meet the specific needs of public health students. Many public health students are nonphysicians and have had little exposure to the moral traditions of medicine. Public health ethics, which can be defined as the identification, analysis, and resolution of ethical problems arising in public health practice and research, has substantially different domains from those of medical ethics. Ethical concerns in public health often relate to the dual obligations of public health professionals to acquire and apply scientific knowledge aimed at restoring and protecting the public's health while respecting individual rights to autonomy [10]. There is frequently a need to balance potential societal benefits against potential risks and harms to individuals and communities, such as intrusions on personal privacy [10, 11]. Other ethical concerns relate to the need to ensure a just distribution of the potential risks and benefits of public health resources [11]. Thus, ethics in public health involves an interplay between protecting the welfare of the individual, as in medicine and nursing, and the public health model of protecting the public welfare [10].

The teaching of public health ethics gets its ultimate justification from its contribution to the public's health and well-being [9]. The desirability of teaching ethics to health professionals rests in the fact that health decision-making involves two components: a technical decision requiring the judicious application of scientific knowledge to health problems, and an ethical component that demands the decision also be ethically justified [9]. This is true in both medicine and public health, although public health professionals are concerned about the health and well-being of groups of individuals and whole communities, rather than the health problems of individual patients as in clinical medicine.

Some might concede the value of public health ethics but argue against its place in the crowded public health curriculum [12]. Given the importance of the subject, however, a few credit hours of classroom time seems easily justifiable [13, 14]. Other critics might argue that the basic moral character of public health students has already been formed by the time they enter graduate school [12]. They might question the value of such instruction if ethics cannot be taught to public health students, or if family and society have not already instilled character and virtues [12]. In order to respond to such criticisms, the attainable objectives of ethics instruction must be realistically considered.

What Are the Attainable Objectives of Instruction in Public Health Ethics?

Although it is true that the basic moral character of public health students has been formed by the time they enter graduate school, evidence from developmental psychology research indicates that personal values and problem-solving strategies continue to evolve well into the second and third decade of life [7, 9, 15]. As noted by Pellegrino et al. [9], the values that students espouse and the strategies that they use for problem-solving continue to change as long as they remain in schools and colleges. Curricula in public health ethics are designed not to improve the moral character of students but rather to provide them with the conceptual abilities and decision-making skills they will need to deal successfully with ethical issues in public health research and practice [7]. In this manner, curricula in public health ethics go beyond simply sensitizing students to ethical problems in public health.

The cognitive aspects of public health ethics that can be taught include the identification of the ethical commitments of public health research and practice, recognition of ethical issues and problems in public health, critical reflection on one's personal values and obligations as a public health professional, knowledge of central concepts such as the elements of informed consent in human subjects research, understanding of important decision-making procedures, and the application of concepts and methods for ethical decision-making to actual cases in public health ethics [7, 12]. The latter involves identification of the relevant principles, rules, duties, or obligations, clarification of conflicts between principles and attempting to resolve such conflicts through further specification, and making and justifying ethical decisions through moral reasoning [7, 9, 12]. An important part of this process is the identification of possible objections to ethical choices and reasons for such objections and the formulation of counterarguments or modification of ethical decisions [9, 12]. Other aspects of ethics that can be taught include a familiarity with the burgeoning literature on public health ethics and the methodology of empirical research studies [7, 12]. The latter often combine the techniques of epidemiology, the social sciences, and ethical analysis [9]. Thus, as Pellegrino argued persuasively from the perspective of a clinical ethicist, there is much to be gained from teaching ethics:

> Ethics can indeed be taught. It is a branch of philosophy, a discipline with its own content and method, as teachable as any other discipline. Ethics, as Aristotle taught, is an eminently practical discipline. It deals with concrete judgments in situations in which action must be taken despite uncertainty . . . . It is hard to see how a discipline that aims to make ethical decisions more orderly, systematic, and rational could be deleterious or how leaving everything to sentiment or feeling could be preferable [12].

Some caution is warranted, however, in projecting the potential benefits of instruction in public health ethics. There is only limited evidence that instruction in ethics makes health professionals and scientists behave more ethically [16]. Improvements in knowledge and cognitive skills do not necessarily translate into desirable behavioral change [16, 17]. Knowledge of what constitutes a real or perceived conflict of interest, for example, does not guarantee one's ability to avoid such conflicts in public health practice or research.

Any attempt to develop curriculum in public health ethics must acknowledge the broader cultural milieu within which ethics instruction must function [17, 18]. A school of public health can be seen as a community with its own culture and subcultures [18]. Public health students are taught what is valued in that culture and provided with opportunities for internalizing these core values. Professional enculturation is a fundamental part of the educational process [17]. Thus, there is a need to balance formal instruction in public health ethics with the informal teaching and mentoring of students. Of course, the process of socialization and exposure to core values in public health may begin well in advance of formal entry into schools of public health [18]. Many public health students are mid-career professionals or members of other health professions.

What Should Guide Curriculum Design?

Curriculum design should take into account the frequency of ethical problems and how often public health professionals must analyze and attempt to resolve them [9]. Ethical problems that are more likely to be encountered in public health research and practice should ideally be featured in public health ethics curricula. The results of recent ethics surveys on practicing public health professionals could serve as a guide to the selection of curricular topics and ethical case studies [19, 20].

Student needs and interests should also guide curriculum design. Our curriculum needs assessment and survey of public health graduate students at Tulane University [1, 3] suggested substantial gaps in the bioethics knowledge of these students. Only about 8% (18 of 236) had ever read any proposed ethics guidelines for epidemiologists. Few of the students were able to identify important developments or concerns in bioethics such as the Nueremberg Code or the principles of beneficence, nonmaleficence, justice, and respect for the autonomy of persons. Only about 19% (46 of 236) of the students surveyed demonstrated knowledge of the ethical significance of the Tuskegee Syphilis Study. There was substantial interest among the students, however, in learning more about ethics in public health and epidemiology. In designing new elective courses on public health ethics, we took into account the fact that Tulane University has many students from the United States who are interested in careers in international health research, former Peace Corps volunteers, and students from other countries. For this reason, we included discussions of ethical issues in cross-cultural research such as alternative theories of informed consent, as well as issues arising in studies of indigenous populations and other vulnerable persons in other parts of the world [2, 3].

Institutional resources and existing linkages are further considerations in curriculum design. Many schools of public health are in close proximity to medical schools or centers for clinical ethics that already offer courses in medical ethics. Other institutional resources include law schools offering courses of instruction in health law. Ethics programs at schools of social work and nursing and departments of human genetics also provide potential resources that ought to be taken into account in designing public health ethics curricula.

What Should Be the Basic Curricular Goals in Public Health Ethics?

Although there are currently no national standards for ethics instruction at schools of public health, ethics courses are offered in at least some public health training programs [2, 4]. These would be the logical starting place for identifying basic curricular goals in public health ethics and developing model curricula. The content of short courses and seminar series on research ethics offered at many academic medical centers in the United States might also facilitate the development of model curricula in public health ethics [6, 21].

At Tulane University, an elective course on "Ethics, Epidemiology, and Public Health Research" was offered for the first time in spring 1995 [2, 3]. Similar courses have been developed at the University of Miami School of Medicine and at the University of South Carolina School of Public Health [4]. In the course offered at Tulane, students learned how to identify and solve ethical problems and conflicts arising in epidemiology and other public health disciplines using methods of ethical decision-making. A combination of lectures and small-group discussions of assigned readings and case studies was used for this purpose. The students were exposed to the burgeoning literature on the ethics of epidemiologic research and practice. The course relied heavily on case studies and assigned readings. An important goal of the course was to discuss cross-cultural differences and perspectives on ethical issues such as theories of informed consent and to identify issues arising in studies of vulnerable persons including children, elderly people, and indigenous populations. Although the emphasis was on epidemiologic research and practice, the lecture materials and assigned readings were general enough to interest students from other departments, such as International Health and Development and Applied Health Sciences.

The curriculum for the course on "Ethics, Epidemiology, and Public Health Research" was developed by first defining the learning objectives, then the evaluation process and how the objectives would be achieved [2, 3]. The case studies and topics for discussion encompassed responsibilities to research subjects, responsibilities to society, responsibilities to employers and funding sources, and responsibilities to professional colleagues. The specific topics covered included a framework for ethics in epidemiology, basic methods of ethical decision-making, ethics guidelines for epidemiologists, privacy and confidentiality protection, issues surrounding informed consent, ethical issues arising in studies of vulnerable populations, ethically optimized observational study designs, the ethics of randomized controlled trials, committee review and the institutional review board system in the United States, communication responsibilities of epidemiologists, issues surrounding the publication and interpretation of research findings, conflicts of interest, the ethics of research sponsorship, and scientific misconduct in epidemiologic research.

The new course was designed to complement an existing course at Tulane University, "Ethical Concerns of Health Managers," without undue overlap [2]. The ethical concerns of health care managers and health policymakers, as discussed in courses currently offered at several universities, include the just allocation of health care resources. As highlighted in a 1985 report on the basic curricular goals in medical ethics [7], the subtopics that could be taught under the general heading of issues in the equitable distribution of health care include:

1. The nature of distributive justice; the responsibilities of the government, health policymakers, patients, and physicians in achieving equity in the distribution of health care; and the effects of the pursuit of equity on the physician's role
2. Patterns of access to health care in the United States and the nature of barriers to adequate health care
3. Alternative models for achieving a more equitable distribution of health care resources
4. The social effects of the different incentives for caregivers that arise in different models of health care organization and funding

The social importance of these topics is indisputable today in this era of health care reform and budgetary constraints. The ethics of managed care [22–24] would logically be included among the basic curricular goals of model curricula in public health ethics, particularly those designed for students enrolled in graduate degree programs in health care administration and health policy. Ethical issues surrounding managed care include the adequacy of patient informed consent and physician disclosures about financial compensation, and physicians' obligations to advocate on behalf of patients who need costly health care services [22–24].

Differences in existing ethics curricula across disciplines as diverse as epidemiology and health care administration underscore the need for flexibility in designing and implementing model curricula in public health. No one curriculum or set of basic curricular goals is likely to meet the needs of all public health disciplines and graduate education programs. This need for flexibility is discussed below along with other challenges to developing and implementing curricula in public health ethics.

What Are Some of the Challenges to Developing and Implementing Curricula in Public Health Ethics?

There are a number of challenges that must be overcome in designing and implementing ethics curricula at schools of public health and other institutions that train public health professionals. One is the diversity of public health disciplines, students, and graduate education programs. The latter include master's degree programs, doctoral programs, and special degree programs such as Doctor of Medicine–Master of Public Health (MD-MPH) joint degree programs. There are also an increasing number of nontraditional degree programs such as certificate training programs and distance-based learning in public health. Public health students also have diverse professional backgrounds, life experiences, and career goals. This diversity of public health students and training programs suggests that no single curriculum in public health ethics is likely to meet the needs of all; flexibility will be required in terms of the number of credit hours of instruction, course content, reading materials, and the like. For example, courses on ethical issues in health care administration or health policy are less likely to be of interest to students pursuing careers in epidemiology or international health research. Public health includes such diverse disciplines as health policy, ethics, epidemiology, the behavioral sciences, health education, health systems management, and environmental sciences.

A further challenge to the design and implementation of public health ethics curricula is the lack of sustained institutional support for such efforts at some institutions. At the World Health Organization–International Society for Environmental Epidemiology–sponsored International Workshop on Ethical and Philosophical Issues in Environmental Epidemiology in North Carolina, attended by epidemiologists and moral philosophers from Europe and the Americas, the workshop participants strongly recommended that professional organizations and institutions invest in programs for epidemiologists to facilitate their ongoing improvement in ethics knowledge and practice [1, 25]. Similar efforts are needed in other public health disciplines.

To a greater or lesser extent, deans and curriculum committee members at schools of public health have tended to overlook the importance of rigorous instruction in ethics. Like medical school administrators in past decades [7], they often seem to have reached the conclusion that "courses in ethics are fine as long as one or more interested faculty members want to teach them, but no deeper institutional commitment needs to be made and no additional resources need to be devoted to a teaching program." Greater institutional support and encouragement from groups such as the ASPH and the Association of Teachers of Preventive Medicine will be needed if enhancements in public health ethics curricula are to be sustained.

There are recent signs that levels of institutional interest in public health ethics instruction are improving. In 1995, for example, "short courses" on ethics and epidemiology were offered for the first time by epidemiology summer programs hosted by the University of Michigan School of Public Health and the New England Epidemiology Institute [2, 4]. Similar elective courses are now offered at other institutions.

The expansion of such efforts will require the additional training and recruitment of faculty qualified to teach courses in public health ethics. Currently, there is a paucity of trained instructors who are knowledgeable about public health ethics. In a survey on epidemiology faculty at United States schools of public health designed to assess the priority placed on the instruction of ethical issues in graduate epidemiology curricula [20], only three respondents (3%) had taught an ethics course during the past 2 years. Sixty (66%) of the faculty who had taught a class during this period, however, indicated that they had included at least some discussion of ethical issues in epidemiology in their course material [20]. Factors that contributed to not addressing ethical issues in all or some courses included "few resource materials available" (23% of respondents); lack of interest in ethical issues was not a major factor [20]. Only one respondent had taken a course in ethical issues in epidemiology as a part of graduate study. In discussing these findings, Rossignol and Goodmonson [20] noted that several faculty who responded to their survey commented that they would like to include more ethics material in their courses but were unaware of published materials. In a recent international ethics survey on environmental epidemiologists [19], 70% of the respondents indicated that they desired to learn more about ethics; 41% indicated that they wished to participate further in the integration of ethics into the research, practice, and teaching of environmental epidemiology [19].

A related challenge to the design and implementation of public health ethics curricula has been the lack of instructional materials tailored specifically to meet the needs of public health students. Texts on research ethics and the ethics of epidemiologic research and practice may help to alleviate this problem [6, 26–28]. There is still a need for further published case studies on public health ethics suitable for teaching purposes, however, including detailed case studies and study questions helpful for teaching ethics to public health students.

Conclusions

Public health students should have some understanding of the concepts and language of ethics and at least a rudimentary understanding of major moral traditions. The tension between Kantian and utilitarian perspectives is a familiar one in public health. It is important for public health students to be skilled at ethical decision-making so that they can appropriately make and justify ethical decisions. They need to be in a position to identify and solve moral problems in their own public health research and practice. Decisions between alternative conceptual or analytical frameworks for ethical analysis ought to take into account practicality and applicability to actual moral problems in public health as well as theoretical considerations [29, 30].

Groups such as the ASPH, the Association of Teachers of Preventive Medicine, and the American College of Epidemiology should play a leadership role in encouraging the development and implementation of model curricula in public health ethics. A logical first step would be to hold a national meeting or workshop with the overall goal of bringing together experts from public health, ethics, and curriculum development to further consider what model curricula in public health ethics might consist of—what steps should be taken to develop them, and how the end products would be implemented and evaluated. Individuals who are currently teaching ethics to public health students could be invited to summarize their course syllabi and teaching experiences. A core group of individuals from various disciplines could then work toward actually producing model curricula in public health ethics. Such curricula would provide national standards for adequate instruction in public health ethics or at least clarify basic curricular goals in this area.

As innovative curricula on ethics are developed for public health students, there will be a need to keep abreast of future refinements in methods for ethical decision-making and improved theoretical foundations [29, 30]. Although little is known now about the impact of ethics instruction on public health practice [1], it is becoming increasingly clear that schools of public health and other institutions that train public health professionals should provide basic instruction in ethics designed to meet the specific needs of public health students.

References

1. Coughlin, S.S., and G.D. Etheredge. On the Need for Ethics Curricula in Epidemiology. *Epidemiology* (1995):6:566–567.
2. Coughlin, S.S., and G.D. Etheredge. Teaching Ethics and Epidemiology: Initial Experiences at Two Schools of Public Health. *Epidemiol Monit* (1995):16:5–7.
3. Coughlin, S.S., G.D. Etheredge, C. Metayer, and S.A. Martin Jr. Curriculum Development in Epidemiology and Ethics at the Tulane School of Public Health and Tropical Medicine. Results of a Needs Assessment and Plans for the Future. Paper presented to the Association of Schools of Public Health Council on Epidemiology, Washington, D.C., October 30, 1994.
4. Goodman, K.W., and R.J. Prineas. Toward an Ethics Curriculum in Epidemiology. In: Coughlin, S.S., and T.L. Beauchamp, editors, *Ethics and Epidemiology*. New York, NY: Oxford University Press (1996).
5. Campbell, C.S., and A.M. Rossignol. Moral Literacy in Epidemiology. *Epidemiol Monit* (1995):16:5–6.
6. Korenman, S.G., and A.C. Shipp. *Teaching the Responsible Conduct of Research Through a Case Study Approach. A Handbook for Instructors*. Washington, D.C.: Association of American Medical Colleges (1994).
7. Culver, C.M., K.D. Clouser, B. Gert, et al. Basic Curricular Goals in Medical Ethics. *N Engl J Med* (1985):312:253–256.
8. Mitchell, K.R., T.J. Lovat, and C.M. Myser. Teaching Bioethics to Medical Students: the Newcastle Experience. *Med Educ* (1992):26:290–300.
9. Pellegrino, E.D., M. Siegler, and P.A. Singler. Teaching Clinical Ethics. *J Clin Ethics* (1990):1:175–180.
10. Lappé, M. Ethics and Public Health. In: Last, J.M., editor, *Maxy–Rosenau Public Health and Preventive Medicine* (12th ed.). Norwalk, CT: Appleton-Century-Crofts (1986):1867–1877.
11. Coughlin, S.S., and T.L. Beauchamp. Ethics, Scientific Validity, and the Design of Epidemiologic Studies. *Epidemiology* (1992):3:343–347.
12. Pellegrino, E.D. Teaching Medical Ethics: Some Persistent Questions and Some Responses. *Acad Med* (1989):64:701–703.
13. Callahan, D., and S. Bok. *Ethics Teaching in Higher Education*. New York, NY: Plenum Press (1980).
14. LaPidus, J.B., and B. Mishkin. Values and Ethics in the Graduate Education of Scientists. In: May, W.W., editor, *Ethics and Higher Education*. New York, NY: Macmillan (1990):238–298.
15. Bok, D.C. Can Ethics Be Taught? *Change* (1976):8:26–30.
16. Arnold, R.M., G.J. Povar, and J.D. Howell. The Humanities, Humanistic Behavior, and the Humane Physician: A Cautionary Note. *Ann Intern Med* (1987):106:313–318.
17. Hafferty, F.W., and R. Franks. The Hidden Curriculum, Ethics Teaching, and the Structure of Medical Education. *Acad Med* (1994):69:861–871.
18. Bloom, S.W. Reform Without Change? Look Beyond the Curriculum (Editorial). *Am J Public Health* (1995):85:907–908.
19. Soskolne, C.L., G.S. Jhangri, B. Hunter, and M. Close. Interim Report on the International Society for Environmental Epidemiology/Global Environmental Epidemiology Network Ethics Survey. Working Paper Presented at the Joint *WHO–ISEE International Workshop on*

Ethical and Philosophical Issues in Environmental Epidemiology. Research Triangle Park, NC, September 16–18, 1994. *J Total Environ* (1996):184:5–11.

20. Rossignol, A.M., and S. Goodmonson. Are Ethical Topics Included in the Graduate Epidemiology Curriculum? *Am J Epidemiol* (1996):142:1265–1268.

21. Sachs, G.A., and M. Siegler. Teaching Scientific Integrity and the Responsible Conduct of Research. *Acad Med* (1993):68:871–875.

22. Annas, G.J. Reframing the Debate on Health Care Reform by Replacing our Metaphors. *N Engl J Med* (1995):332:744–745.

23. Pellegrino, E.D. Ethics. *JAMA* (1994):271:1668–1670.

24. Thomasma, D.C. The Ethics of Managed Care and Cost Control. *Trends Health Care Law Ethics* (1995):10:33–36.

25. World Health Organization Meeting Report. *Joint WHO–ISEE International Workshop on Ethical and Philosophical Issues in Environmental Epidemiology.* Research Triangle Park, NC, September 16–18, 1994. *J Total Environ* (1996):184:131–136.

26. Coughlin, S.S., and T.L. Beauchamp, editors. *Ethics and Epidemiology.* New York, NY: Oxford University Press (1996).

27. Coughlin, S.S., editor. *Ethics in Epidemiology and Clinical Research: Annotated Readings.* Chestnut Hill, MA: Epidemiology Resources Inc. (1995).

28. Penslar, R.I., editor. *Research Ethics. Cases and Materials.* Indianapolis, IN: University of Indiana Press (1995):3–12.

29. Beauchamp, T.L., and J.F. Childress. *Principles of Biomedical Ethics* (4th ed.). New York, NY: Oxford University Press (1994).

30. Beauchamp, T.L. Moral Foundations. In: Coughlin, S.S., and T.L. Beauchamp, editors, *Ethics and Epidemiology.* New York, NY: Oxford University Press (1996).

CHAPTER 9

ETHICS INSTRUCTION AT SCHOOLS OF PUBLIC HEALTH IN THE UNITED STATES

S.S. Coughlin, W. Katz, and D. Mattison

There has been increasing interest in developing curricula on public health ethics and providing instruction on ethics and scientific integrity to students enrolled in public health training programs [1–6]. The Council on Education for Public Health criteria for graduate schools of public health (amended in October 1993) emphasize public health values, concepts, and ethics, although the council does not have specific requirements for ethics instruction. Instruction in health care ethics is an accreditation requirement for graduate training programs in health care administration. Another important development has been the National Institutes of Health mandate for extramural research training programs to provide instruction on scientific integrity and ethical principles in research to trainees [1]. However, relatively little is known about the extent of instruction on public health ethics and the emphasis that is currently placed on ethics and scientific integrity at schools of public health and other institutions that train public health professionals [3, 7–9].

The Association of Schools of Public Health Education Committee undertook a national survey of schools of public health in the United States in early 1996 to determine how they addressed ethical issues in public health. The purpose was to provide a general picture of what presently existed in the way of public health ethics curricula.

Methods

The survey was initiated in January 1996 by sending an explanatory letter with a list of questions for discussion to the deans of the accredited U.S. schools of public health. The letter asked the deans to have at least one individual at their school who "is most knowledgeable about ethics curricula" review the list of questions and complete an ethics survey contact form. Reminders with a second copy of the ethics survey contact form were sent to the deans at the end of January 1996. The questions for discussion with the identified contact person(s) were as follows:

- What ethics courses, graduate degree programs, or continuing professional education are currently being offered?
- Who teaches the course, and what is the teacher's professional background?

"Ethics Instruction at Schools of Public Health in the United States" originally appeared in the American Journal of Public Health (1999):89:768–770. Used with permission of the American Public Health Association.

- Which department or program offers the course?
- Is the course required or is it an elective?
- Which students take the course and how many or what proportion of them take it?
- Is instruction in ethics part of the core curriculum required for all candidates for the master of public health degree?
- Is ethics instruction required for all doctoral students?
- Is there ethics instruction in personal or professional ethics (e.g., sexual harassment, discrimination, cheating in school, and cultural differences in ethical standards)?
- Is there instruction in research ethics or scientific integrity (e.g., data ownership, authorship, and scientific fraud)?
- Is there faculty training or professional development in ethics topics?
- Are there perceived gaps in the current ethics curricula?
- Are short courses, seminar series, or invited lectures on ethics topics offered?
- Are lectures on ethics topics included in other courses such as health law, etc.?
- Are there future plans to develop course work or programs in public health ethics?
- Are there activities that take place outside formal courses that focus on ethics issues?

Information was obtained from roughly half of the schools through telephone interviews or from detailed written responses provided by the contact person.

Results

Interviews were completed for 24 of 28 (86%) of the schools. Of the completed interviews, 13 of 24 (54%) were completed in the winter of 1996 and the remainder (11 of 24, or 46%) were completed in the fall of 1997.

Information was obtained about a large number of ethics courses, graduate degree programs, and continuing professional education currently being offered (results not shown). The professional background of the faculty members who taught these ethics courses included bioethics, biostatistics, environmental health sciences, epidemiology, geriatrics, health behavior and health promotion, health care administration, health services management, health policy, health law, medicine, philosophy, political science, psychology, sociology, and theology.

The department or program that offered these courses included behavioral science or health behavior (3 of 24 surveyed schools); biostatistics (1 school); community health studies (2 schools); epidemiology (3 schools); health management, health services administration, or health policy (14 schools); health law or ethics (2 schools); sociomedical science (1 school); or all of the divisions of the school (1 school).

Instruction on ethics was required for all students at only 1 (4%) of the 24 schools surveyed. An additional 7 schools required ethics instruction for some students. Fourteen schools (58%) offered elective courses on ethics but required no ethics course. Two schools (8%) had no ethics courses.

Most of the schools surveyed (18 of 24, or 75%) offered some instruction in personal or professional ethics (e.g., sexual harassment, discrimination, cheating in school, and cultural differences in ethical standards). There was instruction in research ethics or scientific integrity (e.g., data ownership, authorship, and scientific fraud) at 22 (92%) of the schools.

Only 9 (38%) of the schools offered faculty training or professional development in ethics. This included invited lectures and seminars on various topics, a monthly lunch-time discussion group, a 1-day short course on ethical issues in research and public health, and training and education offered to faculty, at special conferences of their choosing and as part of their own career development.

There were perceived gaps in the ethics curricula at 20 (83%) of the schools. These gaps included the ethics of health policy, scientific integrity, sexual harassment and personal ethics, ethics and epidemiology, and conflicts of interest in industry and in environmental science.

Most of the schools (19 of 24, or 79%) offered short courses, seminar series, or invited lectures on ethical topics, and most (23 of 24, or 96%) included lectures on ethics topics in other courses such as health law. Examples of the latter included lectures on ethics in a course on health maintenance organizations and managed care, discussion of the ethics of AIDS in an AIDS epidemiology course, sessions on ethics in a course on principles of public health, lectures on research ethics in an advanced methods course in epidemiology, and discussion of the ethics of biomonitoring and genetic susceptibility in an environmental health course.

At most of the schools (17 of 24, or 71%) there were activities that took place outside of formal courses on ethics issues. These included student independent research projects on applied ethics, student seminars, nondegree bioethics instruction offered through a university extension, a regional bioethics forum, ethics case conferences, and community settings for class projects and field training that provide opportunities to focus on "real world" ethical issues.

Discussion

The results of this national survey provide information about the extent of formal instruction in public health ethics and scientific integrity at U.S. schools of public health during a period of increased interest in the ethics of public health research and practice. Although these findings indicate that many schools of public health were, at the time of the survey, offering such courses, at least on an elective basis, some graduate programs in public health do not offer or require such instruction.

With respect to the limitations of this survey, coursework and degree requirements are evolving at some schools, and information obtained in 1996 and 1997 may be out of date. Information about ethics instruction may also have been misreported or hard to categorize at some schools. This survey collected only limited information about the content or methods of instruction. It also provided no information about ethics instruction at medical schools, which train about 20% of the public health graduates in the United States (Suzanne Dandoy, December 1997, written communication).

In 1974, Bluestone carried out a survey on the extent and nature of instruction in medical and social ethics by sending a letter and brief questionnaire to the deans of 19 schools of public health in the United States [8]. Results obtained from 15 responding schools indicated that the majority did not offer any studies of the ethical basis of public health practice. Some schools expressed doubt that such a topic could be taught [8]. Others felt that the topic (the ethics of public health programs) was already covered in other courses.

In the mid-1990s, Rossignol and Goodmonson [9] undertook a national survey to assess the priority placed on the instruction of ethical issues in graduate epidemiology curricula by professors of epidemiology in schools of public health in the United States. The responses from 101 faculty members (79% of those queried) indicated that 86% believed that education concerning ethical issues in epidemiological research should be included in the curriculum [9]. Only 3 respondents (3%) had taught an ethics course during the past 2 years, although 60 (66%) of the faculty members who had taught a class during this period indicated that they had included at least some discussion of ethical issues in epidemiology in their course material. The topics most frequently included concerned the protection of human subjects, clinical trials, screening programs, and use or abuse of data [9].

The rationale for teaching ethics to public health students has been previously outlined [1, 2, 4, 6]. Curricula in public health ethics are designed not to improve the moral character of students but rather to provide them with the conceptual abilities and decision-making skills they will need to deal successfully with ethical issues in their own research and practice. The cognitive aspects of ethics that can be taught include identification of the ethical commitments of public health research and practice, recognition of ethical issues and problems, critical reflection on one's personal values and obligations as a public health professional, knowledge of central concepts such as the elements of informed consent, and the application of concepts and methods for ethical decision-making to actual cases in public health ethics [1, 8, 10, 11]. Nevertheless, some caution is warranted in projecting the potential benefits of instruction in public health ethics [12, 13]. Improvements in knowledge and cognitive skills do not necessarily translate into desirable behavioral change.

In summary, the results of the reported survey indicated that training programs at U.S. schools of public health varied greatly in how much attention they gave to ethics instruction. Ethics curricula also varied in their form and content. Although innovation and creativity in training programs are desirable, there were, at the time of the study (or even until now), no national standards for adequate instruction in public health ethics. Model curricula in public health ethics should be developed to help fill this gap [1].

Acknowledgments

The authors thank David Carpenter, Patricia Buffler, and the other members of the Association of Schools of Public Health Education Committee for their assistance with this survey. Andrew Dannenberg and Mila Aroskar provided comments on an earlier version of this manuscript.

References

1. Coughlin, S.S. Model Curricula in Public Health Ethics. *Am J Prev Med* (1996):12:247–251.
2. Coughlin, S.S., and G.D. Etheredge. On the Need for Ethics Curricula in Epidemiology. *Epidemiology* (1995):6:566–567.
3. Coughlin, S.S., G.D. Etheredge, C. Metayer, et al. Remember Tuskegee: Public Health Student Knowledge of the Ethical Significance of the Tuskegee Syphilis Study. *Am J Prev Med* (1996):12:242–246.
4. Coughlin, S.S., C.L. Soskolne, and K.W. Goodman. *Case Studies in Public Health Ethics.* Washington, D.C.: American Public Health Association (1997).

5. Coughlin, S.S. *Ethics in Epidemiology and Public Health Practice: Collected Works.* Columbus, GA: Quill Publications (1997).

6. Goodman, K.W., and R.J. Prineas. Toward an Ethics Curriculum in Epidemiology. In: Coughlin, S.S., and T.L. Beauchamp, editors, *Ethics and Epidemiology.* New York, NY: Oxford University Press (1996).

7. Coughlin, S.S. On the Role of Ethics Committees in Epidemiology Professional Societies. *Am J Epidemiol* (1997):146:209–213.

8. Bluestone, N.R. Teaching of Ethics in Schools of Public Health. *Am J Public Health* (1976):66:478–479.

9. Rossignol, A.M., and S. Goodmonson. Are Ethical Topics in Epidemiology Included in the Graduate Epidemiology Curricula? *Am J Epidemiol* (1995):142:1265–1268.

10. Pellegrino, E.D., M. Siegler, and P.A. Singer. Teaching Clinical Ethics. *J Clin Ethics* (1990):1:175–80.

11. Bok, D.C. Can Ethics Be Taught? *Change* (1976):8:26–30.

12. Arnold, R.M., G.J. Povar, and J.D. Howell. The Humanities, Humanistic Behavior, and the Humane Physician: a Cautionary Note. *Ann Intern Med* (1987):106:313–318.

13. Bloom, S.W. Reform Without Change? Look Beyond the Curriculum (Editorial). *Am J Public Health* (1995):85:907–908.

CHAPTER 10

USING CASES WITH CONTRARY FACTUAL INFORMATION TO ILLUSTRATE AND FACILITATE ETHICAL ANALYSIS

Steven S. Coughlin

Introduction

There has been increasing interest in developing practical, nontheoretical tools for analyzing ethical problems in public health, biomedicine, and other scientific disciplines, so that students and practicing health professionals and researchers can make and justify ethical decisions. The role of ethical decision-making in public health and biomedical research is often to identify and analyze instances of ethical conflict or uncertainty, with the goal of making sound decisions upon which to act. There is often a need to negotiate or resolve ethical conflicts or disagreements with attention to the rights, responsibilities, and interests of the parties involved.

Tools for ethical decision-making, together with case studies on ethics, are often used in the classroom both in graduate education programs and in continuing professional education [1–4]. Group discussion of ethics case studies is an important instructional method in ethics [5–7]. Ethical awareness and ethical sensitivity are practiced skills [8], and students can benefit from opportunities to further develop their analytical skills, to recognize ethical issues, to address moral ambiguity, and to stimulate their moral imagination [3–9].

This essay provides a practical approach for illustrating and facilitating ethical analysis using cases with contrary facts and circumstances. This tool for ethical analysis is intended to complement rather than replace theoretical approaches to moral reasoning. As discussed below, the potential applications of this approach include its use in the classroom and in research and practice in a variety of professional fields and scientific disciplines.

Background

Several approaches for ethical analysis have been proposed for use in medical and public health research and practice. These include the principle-based approach of Beauchamp and Childress [10], case-based or analogical methods such as casuistry [11, 12], and moral rule–based systems [13, 14]. Other approaches depend on rights-based theories, duty-based

"Using Cases With Contrary Factual Information to Illustrate and Facilitate Ethical Analysis" originally appeared in *Science and Engineering Ethics (2008):14:103–110*. Used with kind permission of Springer Science and Business Media.

theories, contractarianism, virtue ethics, the ethics of care, and communitarianism. For example, in humanitarian approaches to health care ethics, people respond to human suffering and realize human fulfillment by acting in a virtuous manner based on compassion or altruism [15]. Because it is impractical for the vast majority of health professionals to master such diverse theoretical frameworks in order to identify and resolve ethical problems in their own research or practice, nontheoretical or practical steps for identifying and analyzing ethical issues have also been proposed.

From a practical standpoint, Beauchamp [16] noted that ethical problems can sometimes be resolved by obtaining further facts about matters at the center of the controversy or by more clearly defining the language used by the disputing parties. Disagreement about facts can often be resolved by appeal to objective data. Other steps that can be taken to resolve ethical controversies include the use of examples and counterexamples and accompanying analysis of the arguments to expose their inadequacies, gaps, and fallacies. In addition, ethical problems can sometimes be resolved by encouraging the disputing parties to adopt a new policy or code, such as ethical guidelines, professional ethical norms, and standards of practice [16].

Other authors have observed that practical steps in ethical decision-making begin with assessing the available factual information, identifying the relevant ethical issues or questions, identifying the stakeholders and values at stake, and identifying the available options including possible alternative courses of action [2, 3, 17]. The remaining steps include selecting the best alternative supported by this analysis and evaluating the actions taken and their eventual outcomes.

Cases with Contrary Facts or Circumstances

Cases with contrary facts and circumstances are a potentially useful tool for illustrating and facilitating ethical analysis, including in classroom settings. Such ethics cases are composed in two or more alternative ways so that the facts, circumstances, or framing of one version runs counter to that of the other version(s). The cases may be fictional or nonfictional. The use of cases with contrary facts, as discussed in this essay, is different from the concept of *counterfactual claims* in philosophy and logic (although, both the philosophic concept of counterfactual claims and the idea of contrary facts require critical thinking for application). Claims are central to philosophy and are referred to as counterfactual claims when they are phrased in the negative, for example, some philosophers have claimed that the immortality of the soul cannot be deduced through reason alone. Every claim implies a counterfactual claim. In contrast, the practical approach for ethical analysis proposed in this essay focuses on alternative versions of cases that are written and framed in different ways so that alternative perspectives are emphasized. The alternative versions of each case are intended to arouse the interest of the audience (e.g., students in a scientific or biomedical training program), to have educational value, and to have application beyond the particulars of the case. This approach is likely to be useful for helping students and practicing scientists and health professionals consider ethical problems from different perspectives and identify the relevant and perhaps distinct ethical issues or questions arising from those perspectives. A growing literature has focused on the use of case materials for ethics instruction in a variety of health professions and scientific disciplines [1–4, 6, 7, 18]. Case-study methods in general are particularly well suited for learning situations where the issues are not clear-cut and contain some ambiguity [4]. As noted by Howard and colleagues [4]:

A number of considerations are relevant to the development of individual case studies. Similar to a good storyteller, an effective case study tells a story that arouses the interest of the audience because it presents characters and situations that hold personal relevance or are likely to elicit empathy. Second, it has pedagogic value [and] should serve some educational function. Third, the case study should be conflict provoking or provocative and force some decision making. Fourth, the case should have generality; that is, principles derived from particulars of the case should have greater utility and applicability to the general content area of the discipline. ([4], p. 151)

Other authors have also detailed approaches for leading an ethics discussion using case study materials [2, 3]. As Jennings ([3], p. 6) explains, "The key to any successful group discussion of ethical questions lies in the skill of the facilitator who guides the discussion and in the curiosity and engagement of the participants. They must open their minds to unfamiliar ideas and learn to see connections between the decision, actions, and their consequences for the person, for others, and for society as a whole." For a discussion of ethics to succeed, he argues that it is important to overcome "a sense of powerlessness and alienation—the feeling that nothing one does as an individual really makes any difference." Jennings ([3], p. 7) further notes, "When you feel helpless you are not prone to accept the idea that you have responsibility for what happens to you or for what goes on in society . . . . The trick is to make connections between the *big issues* and more tangible, controllable aspects of personal life, and to lead the discussion beyond the classroom by considering ways participants can get involved in community activities and address some of the problems discussed in class."

These explications of approaches for leading a discussion of ethics using case-study materials naturally leads into a discussion of how cases with contrary facts can be useful for illustrating and facilitating ethical analysis.

Example of How Cases with Contrary Facts can be Useful for Illustrating and Facilitating Ethical Analysis

As an example of how cases with contrary facts can be useful for ethical analysis, two versions of a case are presented below that focus on humanitarian concerns shared by many professionals in scientific, biomedical, and public health disciplines. Like others in society, health professionals, biomedical researchers, and other scientists often choose their career path because of their desire to contribute meaningfully to the public good. For this reason, the following case is designed to appeal to those humanitarian interests.

Case for Graduate Students in Public Health, Biomedicine, or Scientific Research

Results from a recent cross-sectional survey suggested that 86% of North Americans believe that the actions of one person can have an impact in the world, and that many people in the general population hope to make a positive impact. It seems likely that many individuals in a variety of health professions and scientific disciplines also hope to have a positive influence/effect on society, perhaps by making important scientific or medical discoveries, preventing disease, or helping people to build secure, productive, and healthy communities. Indeed, alleviating human suffering and helping people to reach their potential are among the humanitarian aims of a large number of private organizations (e.g., Doctors Without Borders, Project HOPE, MercyCorps, and CARE) and government agencies such as the World Health Organization and the United Nations Educational, Scientific, and Cultural Organization [19]. Should longitudinal studies of students enrolled in health and scientific training programs be conducted to identify predictors of which students will go on to make a difference in the world? If so, should the longitudinal studies be observational or have a randomized intervention to increase the likelihood that students might make an especially valuable contribution?

These statements raise a number of important ethical and social issues that might not be readily apparent from this simple description. For example, questions could be raised about whether it would be desirable to undertake a study to determine characteristics of students that predict whether they will actually make a difference in the world. And, if undertaking such research were desirable, what type of study design would be appropriate? To address such questions and identify and resolve conflicts in values and ethical considerations, practical steps for ethical analysis could be followed. For example, professional ethical norms and standards of practice could be considered such as those that have bearing on the identification of research questions, choices of study designs, and the like. It might also be helpful to assess the available factual information, identify the relevant ethical issues or questions, and identify the stakeholders and values involved.

To see how the use of cases with contrary facts can facilitate such efforts, consider the following alternative (fictional) versions of this case, which include hypothetical developments and which are composed in two very different ways so that the framing of the first version runs counter to that of the second.

Version 1

People in a variety of health and scientific disciplines may choose their career path because of their desire to help others in their community and in the world, and to contribute meaningfully to the public good. But can one scientist or health researcher truly make a difference? To identify effective approaches for encouraging students enrolled in health and scientific training programs to do so, a researcher proposed undertaking a controlled trial of a behavioral intervention in which some students would be randomized to a "usual care" comparison group and others to an intervention group, and then followed over time to examine the effectiveness of the intervention in helping students make a positive impact. Soon after the proposed study was announced, a lively discussion ensued about the extent to which the study would adequately respect the intrinsic worth of each student. It was noted that every person is important and can contribute something useful to others. Also, people hold different values and beliefs about what constitutes a positive impact or significant contribution, and the values and beliefs held by the researcher are not necessarily shared by others. Rather than randomizing some students to a "usual care" control group and simply observing them over time, some commentators felt it would be better if the researcher helped to empower all of the students (e.g., through the use of educational counseling, coaching, or other intervention approaches). However, the researcher argued that by gathering scientifically valid information about predictors of especially influential students, the study itself would make an important contribution to society. He felt that it would be inappropriate to use a less rigorous study design.

Now consider the following version of this case with hypothetical developments, which has been rewritten and framed in a very different fashion so that alternative perspectives are emphasized:

Version 2

People in a variety of health and scientific disciplines may choose their career path because of their desire to help others in their community and in the world, and to contribute meaningfully to the public good. But can one scientist or health researcher truly make a difference? To determine predictors of whether a student enrolled in health and scientific training programs will do so, a researcher proposed undertaking a longitudinal study with an observational design. Soon after the proposed study was announced, a heated controversy arose over whether the study was ethical. Critics charged that the proposed study was unethical because it would not adequately respect the intrinsic worth of each student. They argued that every person is important and can contribute something useful to others. Other commentators felt that it would be wrong to study people over time, to see whether they made a contribution to society/the global community, without intervening in some way to help them. From this point of view, it was the observational nature of the study that was objectionable. To fulfill his ethical obligations to the participants, these commentators felt the researcher should help empower the students (e.g., through the use of educational counseling, coaching, or other intervention approaches). In attempting to defend the proposed study, the researcher noted that by gathering scientifically valid information about predictors of especially influential students, the study itself would make an important contribution to society. He felt that it would be unethical to develop and administer an intervention because he felt that his values and beliefs are not necessarily shared by others.

By reading and reflecting on both versions of this fictional case, including hypothetical developments framed in different ways, it is possible to identify several relevant ethical issues or questions, and to assess the available options and possible alternative courses of action from different perspectives. In a class discussion, this is likely to require the help of the instructor or other trained facilitator for the group discussion. Although reasonable people might reach different conclusions about some aspects of this case, several areas of agreement or consensus can be identified. For example, there is broad agreement that every person is important and can contribute something useful. It also appears likely that people may hold different values and beliefs about what constitutes making an important difference, and that alternative scientific approaches for better understanding such questions have certain advantages and disadvantages.

Discussion

Reflection upon cases with contrary facts can help with the analysis of ethical issues including the selection of alternative courses of action and the evaluation of actions that may be taken and their possible outcomes. Of particular interest is the potential use of this method in the classroom, both in graduate education and in continuing professional education courses. The alternative versions of the cases presented in this essay were written and framed so that the narratives would hopefully interest health professionals and scientists who strive to make humanitarian contributions such as important scientific or medical discoveries, preventing disease, or helping people to build better communities.

The development and use of cases with contrary facts and circumstances is likely to be useful for helping students and practicing health professionals and scientists further develop their ethical awareness and ethical sensitivity. The use of the term *ethical sensitivity* in this context should not be taken to imply that the use of cases with contrary facts is modeled after comprehensive frameworks for understanding moral development such as Rest's four-component model of moral behavior, which addresses moral judgment, moral sensitivity, moral motivation, and moral character [8, 20]. Rather, ethical sensitivity in this context refers to an enhanced ability of students and practicing health professionals and scientists to recognize ethical issues and to discern what should be done in particular instances of ethical conflict.

Additional efforts are needed to identify tools for illustrating and facilitating ethical analysis in public health, biomedical research, and clinical medicine [3, 5, 21, 22]. It is important for professionals in public health and medicine to be skilled at ethical decision-making so that they can appropriately make ethical decisions and act responsibly. They need to be in a position to identify and solve ethical problems in their own research and practice. Decisions between alternative analytical approaches for ethical analysis should take into account not only theoretical considerations but also practicality and applicability to actual ethical problems in public health and medicine. Students and practicing scientists and health professionals have a sense of moral discernment and responsibility that can be enhanced and refined through continuing education efforts [4, 8]. One of the hallmarks of ethics instruction in public health and medicine has been innovation and creativity, and this includes developments in case study materials and narrative ethics [1, 3]. Cases with contrary facts, together with practical steps for identifying and analyzing ethical issues, are likely to be useful tools for illustrating and facilitating ethics analysis and stimulating the moral imagination.

References

1. Coughlin, S.S., C.L. Soskolne, and K.W. Goodman. Case Analysis and Moral Reasoning. In: Coughlin, S.S., C.L. Soskolne, and K.W. Goodman, editors, *Case Studies in Public Health Ethics*. Washington, D.C.: American Public Health Association (1997):1–18.
2. Heitman, E. Using Cases in the Study of Ethics. In: Bulger, R.F., E. Heitman, and S.J. Reiser, editors, *The Ethical Dimensions of the Biological and Health Sciences* (2nd ed.). New York, NY: Cambridge University Press (2002):349–364.
3. Jennings, B. Introduction: A Strategy for Discussing Ethical Issues in Public Health. In *Association of Schools of Public Health. Ethics and Public Health: Model Curriculum* (2003):1–12. Available at http://www.asph.org/document.cfm?page=782. Accessed 28 July 2006.
4. Howard, D.E., C. Lothen-Kline, and B.O. Boekeloo. Using the Case-Study Methodology to Teach Ethics to Public Health Students. *Health Promot Pract* (2004):5:151–159.
5. Soskolne, C.L., and L.E. Sieswerda. Implementing Ethics in the Professions: Examples from Environmental Epidemiology. *Sci Total Environ* (2003):9:181–190.
6. Herkert, J.R. Ways of Thinking About and Teaching Ethical Problem Solving: Microethics and Macroethics in Engineering. *Sci Eng Ethics* (2005):11:373–385.
7. Lozano, J.F., G. Palau-Salvador, V. Gozalvez, and A. Boni. The Use of Moral Dilemmas for Teaching Agricultural Engineers. *Sci Eng Ethics* (2006):12:327–334.
8. Rest, J.R. Background: Theory and Research. In: Rest, J.R., and D. Narvaez, editors, *Moral Development in the Professions: Psychology and Applied Ethics*. Hillsdale, NJ: Lawrence Erlbaum Associates (1994):1–26.

9. Callahan, D., and S. Bok, editors. *Ethics Teaching in Higher Education.* New York, NY: Plenum Press (1980).

10. Beauchamp, T.L., and J.F. Childress. *Principles of Biomedical Ethics* (5th ed.) New York, NY: Oxford University Press (2001).

11. Jonsen, A.R., and S.E. Toulmin. *The Abuse of Casuistry.* Berkeley, CA: University of California Press (1988).

12. Arras, J.D. Principles and Particularity: The Role of Cases in Bioethics. *Indiana Law J* (1994):69:983–1014.

13. Clouser, K.D. Common Morality as an Alternative to Principlism. *Kennedy Inst Ethics J* (1995):5:219–236.

14. Gert, B. Making the Morally Relevant Features Explicit: A Response to Carson Strong. *Kennedy Inst Ethics J* (2006):16:59–71.

15. Alkire, S., and L. Chen. Global Health and Moral Values. *Br Med J* (2004):364:1069–1074.

16. Beauchamp, T.L. Moral Foundations. In: Coughlin, S.S., and T.L. Beauchamp, editors, *Ethics and Epidemiology.* New York, NY: Oxford University Press (1996):24–52.

17. Swazey, J., and S.J. Bird. Teaching and Learning Research Ethics. In: Elliott, D., and J.E. Stern, editors, *Research Ethics: A Reader.* Hanover, NH: University Press of New England (1997):1–19.

18. Pimple, K.D. General Issues in Teaching Research Ethics. In: Penslar, R.L., editor, *Research Ethics. Cases and Materials.* Bloomington, IN: Indiana University Press (1995):3–12.

19. ten Have, H., and W.T. Ang. UNESCO's Global Ethics Observatory. *J Med Ethics* (2007):33:15–16.

20. Bebeau, M.J., J.R. Rest, and D. Narvaez. Beyond the Promise: A Perspective on Research in Moral Education. *Educ Res* (1999):28:18–26.

21. Coughlin, S.S. Model Curricula in Public Health Ethics. *Am J Prev Med* (1996):12:247–251.

22. Pellegrino, E.D. Teaching Medical Ethics: Some Persistent Questions and Some Responses. *Acad Med* (1989):64:701–703.

PART V

ETHICS GUIDELINES FOR EPIDEMIOLOGISTS

T he selected reading included in this section discusses the rationale for developing a new set of ethics guidelines for epidemiologists in North America, and includes the ethics guidelines developed for members of the American College of Epidemiology (ACE). The ACE ethics guidelines are indebted to earlier versions of ethics guidelines for epidemiologists such as those drafted for the Industrial Epidemiology Forum and the International Society for Environmental Epidemiology (ISEE). Ethics surveys of epidemiologists belonging to ACE and ISEE also played an important role in identifying core values in the field and helping to lay the groundwork for the development of ethics guidelines for epidemiologists. Following the development of the ACE ethics guidelines, articles by Robert Mckeown, Douglas Weed, and others examined the process by which the ACE ethics guidelines are being disseminated, and further clarified the professional roles and responsibilities of epidemiologists.

Another important development in the past decade was the completion of a set of Principles of the Ethical Practice of Public Health by the Public Health Leadership Society (PHLS) in 2002, which have been adopted by the American Public Health Association and other public health organizations. The Principles of the Ethical Practice of Public Health includes a preamble, a statement of values and beliefs that underlie the code, an explanation of the rationale for a public health code of ethics, notes on the 12 individual ethical principles highlighted in the code, and an explanation of how the principles relate to 12 essential public health services. The preamble states that the code is neither a new nor an exhaustive system of health ethics and that it is primarily intended for public and other institutions in the United States that have a public health mission. Values and beliefs underlying the code include the belief that humans have a right to the resources necessary for health, that humans are inherently social and interdependent, that the effectiveness of institutions depends heavily on the public's trust, that collaboration is a key element to public health, that people and their environment are interdependent, and that each person in a community should have an opportunity to contribute to public discourse. Some of the 12 principles enumerated in the code (e.g., public health should advocate and work for the empowerment of disenfranchised community members, public health institutions should act in a timely manner on the information they have, and they should protect the confidentiality of information that can bring harm to an individual or community if made public) have a direct relation to ethical rules set forth in ethics guidelines for epidemiologists.

Jacquelyn Slomka, in a recent article on professionalism and ethics in public health [1], noted that the PHLS code of ethics is included in professionalism competencies for Master of Public Health (MPH) students that were developed by the Association of Schools of

Public Health (ASPH). The ASPH competencies also state that it is important for MPH students to promote high standards of personal and organizational integrity, compassion, honesty, and respect for all people.

1. Slomka, J., B. Quill, M. desVignes-Kendrick, L.E. Lloyd. Professionalism and Ethics in the Public Health Curriculum. *Public Health Rep* (2008):123 Suppl 2:27–35.

CHAPTER 11

NEW ETHICS GUIDELINES FOR EPIDEMIOLOGY: BACKGROUND AND RATIONALE

D.L. Weed and S.S. Coughlin

Introduction

Nearly a decade has passed since epidemiologists, ethicists, and legal scholars began concerted efforts to write professional ethics guidelines for epidemiologists [1–3]. During this time, guidelines have been prepared by the Industrial Epidemiology Forum (IEF) in 1989 [4], the Council for International Organizations of Medical Sciences (CIOMS) in 1990 [5], the International Epidemiological Association (IEA) in 1990 [6], and for the International Society for Environmental Epidemiology (ISEE) in 1996 [7]. Recently, the American College of Epidemiology (ACE) asked its Ethics and Standards of Practice Committee to produce ethics guidelines [8]. In this commentary, we provide the context and rationale for such an effort, describe the purpose and content of guidelines, and discuss their strengths and weaknesses.

Why Write Another Set of Guidelines?

Perhaps the most obvious reason for a new set of guidelines is that the organization has not developed its own, although ACE members hardly practice in an ethical void. They are guided by other guidelines [4–7], recent books on ethics in epidemiology [9, 10], a growing number of journal articles, and formal courses [11]. A more compelling reason for writing new guidelines is that three issues central to the mission of ACE—education, policy, and advocacy—are inadequately considered in existing ethics guidelines. Ethics education in graduate training programs for epidemiologists or as part of continuing professional education is barely addressed in existing guidelines. Ethical issues concerning the important role of epidemiology in health policy are also inadequately discussed. For the issue of public health advocacy, existing guidelines provide inconsistent recommendations on the extent to which epidemiologists should engage in this aspect of professional practice [12]. Finally, existing guidelines focus more on the equitable distribution of the burdens of research than on the equally important notion of the just distribution of research [13].

A further reason for revisiting and refining existing guidelines is that issues arising in subspecialty areas of epidemiology are inadequately addressed. For example, the guidelines do not address issues that can arise in molecular epidemiology such as those surrounding

"New Ethics Guidelines for Epidemiology: Background and Rationale" originally appeared in Annals of Epidemiology (1999):9:277–280. Used with permission of Elsevier Inc.

the use of banked biological specimens for DNA testing [14] and those concerning biomarkers [15]. Existing guidelines also do not deal adequately with ethical issues arising in field epidemiology and other areas of public health practice such as outbreak investigations, surveillance systems, and evaluation studies [16]. In addition, a reexamination of the issues of privacy, confidentiality, and data security may be warranted in this age of enhanced information technologies.

Beyond these practical reasons lies another justification for new ethics guidelines. These are not static guidelines. As the needs and values of professionals change, so should the guidelines to reflect the changing roles of epidemiologists in society [17]. Epidemiology has undergone increasing scrutiny from the media and from the courts. Likewise, epidemiologists are increasingly challenged by their new-found relationships with regulatory bodies, the legal profession, and employers, such as managed care organizations. Dynamic guidelines require occasional updating and revisiting [18]. Still, the framers may find good reason to reaffirm core values, principles, and rules of professional conduct that may remain relevant because they are rooted in a common morality such as the universal precept of "truth-telling," accepted by all moral persons in all moral traditions. In this context, universal does not mean absolute. Even a universally accepted ethical rule may have exceptions, especially when it conflicts with some other such rule [19].

The Purpose of Guidelines

New guidelines may serve to further define and legitimize the profession of epidemiology. Indeed, guidelines serve the same purpose for any profession [17], each of which is characterized by a specialized body of knowledge and skills, by lengthy education and training, and by the services it provides. Professions are autonomous and self-regulating bodies that profess, that is, affirm their willingness as learned practitioners of their discipline, to provide services. Just as physicians profess (or declare publicly) to treat illness in patients and teachers pledge to educate students, so epidemiologists profess to prevent disease in populations through studying the distribution and determinants of disease and applying that knowledge for the public's benefit [12]. The knowledge required to meet epidemiology's commitment to society through science and public health is broadly conceived and supported by theory, methodology, and practical experience in research and practice. Education and training programs in epidemiology, which are now widely recognized and proliferating, are correspondingly broad and deep. In sum, epidemiology is a profession as the ACE explicitly recognizes. A new set of ethics guidelines may underscore the ACE's commitment to that idea.

It follows that ethics guidelines also alert the public (including employers of epidemiologists) to what they may and may not expect from a professional epidemiologist. Nevertheless, the primary users of a new set of ethics guidelines are the epidemiologists themselves, who are provided with a general description of the moral aspects of their work as well as a guide to moral decision-making in cases of moral uncertainty [20].

The Content of Guidelines

We draw a distinction between moral (i.e., ethics) guidelines, which address a range of general professional obligations, and what Spicer [17] calls "quasi-moral" guidelines, or rules of etiquette for professionals. The latter emphasize procedural matters, such as the proper procedures for consultations or the process for adjudicating disputes. We also recognize the importance of guidelines for good scientific practices within epidemiology, although such guidelines do not focus specifically on the ethics of epidemiologic research. Nevertheless, there is a close relationship between good epidemiology practices and ethical norms in the field (e.g., having a written protocol and submitting that protocol to an independent committee for ethical review).

We also draw a distinction between ethics guidelines and more specific policy statements that have sometimes been drafted by professional societies and consensus committees. For example, a working group formed by the National Institutes of Health and the Centers for Disease Control and Prevention offered specific recommendations for the use of repository materials (e.g., DNA obtained from banked tissues, blood, or other biological specimens) for genetic testing, such as when requirements to obtain the informed consent of subjects can be waived [14]. Additional policy statements of interest to molecular and genetic epidemiologists have been drafted by groups such as the American Society for Human Genetics [21] and the American College of Medical Genetics [22]. Like the more general ethics guidelines, such policy statements on specific issues concerning human subjects need to be periodically revisited and revised, in part because of the rapid advance of scientific technology in molecular genetics and other fields.

We focus here on ethics guidelines, and in this section consider their basic components: core values, duties, and virtues. Core values are the central objectives of the profession of epidemiology, reflecting what the profession stands for and promotes through its work [7]. Duties are those obligations epidemiologists hold to various parties, whether broadly or specifically conceived. Obligations and their implications have been emphasized in published guidelines. Virtues can also be considered a component of ethics guidelines [17]. Virtues—such as honesty, prudence, integrity, and truthfulness—are distinct from core values and obligations. Virtues reflect issues of character for professionals and are important in all aspects of professional practice, including our willingness to use ethics guidelines in everyday professional activities [23]. Although good character does not ensure good conduct (as defined in the existing guidelines), it does affect the ways in which epidemiologists are perceived by society and forms the moral basis of the motivation of professional practitioners to use the guidelines.

What Guidelines Can and Cannot Do

The strength of guidelines is that they not only maintain, promote, and protect professional prestige, but also provide a foundation for the discussion of specific ethical issues in the classroom and in professional practice [1]. When faced with an ethical dilemma, or to some other ethical conflict or challenge, a practitioner may refer to guidelines for general guidance in decision-making. Specific answers to discrete ethical questions, however, should not be expected from any set of guidelines; they are not typically structured to consider the complexity and richness of detail that comprise everyday decision-making at the level of specific cases such as those found in a recent text [24].

Guidelines do not provide the final word on ethical issues; as noted above, they are rather general discussions. Moreover, they do not provide an organizational framework, such as policies and procedures, for dealing with ethics violations. Rather, they can be considered the standard of practice regarding general ethics issues. Specific decisions in particular cases will involve reflection and judgment [19].

Existing Ethics Guidelines in Epidemiology

The events that led to the development of ethics guidelines for epidemiologists have been reviewed elsewhere [1]. Descriptions of the four sets of guidelines that are currently available to professional epidemiologists follow. These have appeared in various publications in a six-year window from 1990 through 1995.

IEF Guidelines

These guidelines emphasize the obligations of epidemiologists to four distinct groups: research subjects, society, funding agencies and employers, and professional colleagues. For example, obligations to research subjects include: protecting their welfare, obtaining informed consent, protecting privacy, maintaining confidentiality, and reviewing research protocols. Obligations to society include: avoiding conflicting interests, avoiding partiality, widening the scope of epidemiology, pursuing responsibilities with due diligence, and maintaining public confidence. Obligations to funders and employers as well as those to colleagues are similarly specified. The IEF guidelines also contain commentary sections on the nature and purpose of guidelines and a detailed discussion of specific components of each general obligation. In addition, the moral foundation of the guidelines is briefly described, which relies primarily (but not exclusively) on four principles of bioethics: autonomy, nonmaleficence, beneficence, and justice. Other principles that are relevant for making moral judgments are acknowledged, including fidelity and conscientiousness. Finally, the authors of these guidelines note that the nature and goals of epidemiology—that is, the core values—are inadequately addressed. Virtues are not mentioned. In sum, the IEF guidelines primarily provide a detailed (and well-organized) description and discussion of professional obligations.

IEA Guidelines

Ethics guidelines drafted by the IEA were never officially adopted and are only available in draft form. They are organized around nine basic points: the first two discuss the definition and purposes of epidemiology and the nature and (core) values of epidemiology. These are followed by a section on basic principles of biomedical ethics—autonomy, beneficence, nonmaleficence, and justice—which also mentions the Helsinki Declaration. The next three sections discuss obligations to individuals, obligations to communities, and access to information. The last sections discuss scientific integrity, professional standards, and cultural variations in values. Virtues are not mentioned. A paragraph on education and training is provided under the heading of professional standards. In sum, the IEA guidelines are rather brief and appear to be a draft document to be used as a starting point for discussion.

CIOMS Guidelines

Like the IEF and IEA guidelines, the CIOMS guidelines were intended to provide a guide to help those who have to deal with ethical issues that arise in epidemiology. Unlike the IEF and IEA guidelines, the CIOMS guidelines are not obligation-based. Rather, they emphasize the review of epidemiological studies; a prominent section describes cross-sectional, case-control, cohort, and experimental study designs. The structure of the guidelines is based on the (same) four principles of bioethics applied to epidemiological studies and uses the following major subheadings: informed consent, maximizing benefit, minimizing harm, confidentiality, and conflict of interests. The final section of the guidelines is a discussion of ethical review procedures.

ISEE Guidelines

These guidelines were prepared for the ISEE. They are based directly on the IEF guidelines and even use the precise language of the earlier effort. The authors of the ISEE guidelines add core values and a definition of environmental epidemiology. They also provide additional components to the general obligations featured in the original IEF guidelines. For example, under the obligation to colleagues, the IEF guidelines proposed the following components: reporting methods and results, confronting unacceptable behavior and conditions, and communicating ethical requirements. To these, the ISEE guidelines added the following: publishing methods and results. It should be noted, however, that issues in publication were also addressed in the commentary section of the IEF guidelines.

Conclusions

From our review of the nature and scope of existing ethics guidelines for epidemiologists, we conclude that an effort to provide a new set of guidelines under the auspices of the ACE is reasonable and warranted. Beyond the idea that it is important to revisit ethics guidelines periodically because professional values and needs change with time, our reasons include the fact that existing guidelines do not carefully examine nor clearly state the obligations and components of obligations involved in three areas central to the ACE: education, policy, and advocacy. Another reason for composing a new set of ethics guidelines is that no current set addresses the topic of professional character (i.e., virtues). Finally, it is not clear the extent to which the concerns and needs of the members of the profession were considered in drafting some of these guidelines; the ISEE guidelines, however, were informed by an international survey of environmental scientists.

Our concerns should not be construed as critical of the framers of previous guidelines nor of the documents themselves. We fully appreciate the effort that was expended to create the existing guidelines and the accompanying commentary. We also understand that other groups such as the Italian Epidemiological Association have undertaken efforts to develop new or refined sets of ethics guidelines. All guidelines remain important, even vital, milestones in epidemiology's search for its ethical foundations.

We look forward to meeting the needs of the ACE with a new set of ethics guidelines for the profession.

Acknowledgments

The comments, suggestions, and encouragement received from Drs. John Andrews, Germaine Buck, Robert McKeown, Rosanne McTyre, Colin Soskolne, Dixie Snider, Michael Bracken, and Sally Vernon are greatly appreciated.

References

1. Soskolne, C.L. Epidemiology: Questions of Science, Ethics, Morality, and Law. *Am J Epidemiol* (1989):129:1–18.

2. MacMahon, B. A Code of Ethical Conduct for Epidemiologists? *J Clin Epidemiol* (1991):44 (I Suppl):147S–149S.

3. Last, J. Professional Standards of Conduct for Epidemiologists. In: Coughlin, S.S., and T.L. Beauchamp, editors, *Ethics and Epidemiology*. New York, NY: Oxford University Press (1996): 53–75.

4. Beauchamp, T.L., R.R. Cook, W.E. Fayerweather, et al. Ethical Guidelines for Epidemiologists. *J Clin Epidemiol* (1991):44 (I Suppl):151S–169S.

5. Bankowski, Z., J.H. Bryant, and J.M. Last, editors. Ethics and Epidemiology: International Guidelines. *Proceedings of the XXVth CIOMS Conference*, November 7–9, 1990. Geneva: CIOMS (1991):137–42.

6. *International Epidemiological Association Guidelines on Ethics for Epidemiologists*. Washington, D.C.: Epidemiology Section Newsletter (Winter 1990).

7. Soskolne, C.L., and A. Light. Towards Ethics Guidelines for Environmental Epidemiologists. *Sci Total Environ* (1996):184:137–147.

8. Coughlin, S.S. On the Role of Ethics Committees in Epidemiology Professional Societies. *Am J Epidemiol* (1997):146:209–213.

9. Coughlin, S.S., editor. *Ethics in Epidemiology and Clinical Research.* Newton, MA: Epidemiology Resources Inc. (1995).

10. Coughlin, S.S., and T.L. Beauchamp, editors. *Ethics and Epidemiology*. New York, NY: Oxford University Press (1996).

11. Goodman, K.W., and R.J. Prineas. Toward an Ethics Curriculum in Epidemiology. In: Coughlin, S.S., and T.L. Beauchamp, editors, *Ethics and Epidemiology*. New York, NY: Oxford (1996):290–303.

12. Weed, D.L. Science, Ethics Guidelines, and Advocacy in Epidemiology. *Ann Epidemiol* (1994):4:166–171.

13. Coughlin, S.S. Environmental Justice: the Role of Epidemiologists in Protecting Unempowered Communities from Environmental Hazards. *Sci Total Environ* (1996):184:67–76.

14. Clayton, E.W., K.K. Steinberg, M.J. Khoury, et al. Informed Consent for Genetic Research on Stored Tissue Samples. *JAMA* (1995):274:1786–1792.

15. Soskolne, C.L. Ethical, Social, and Legal Issues Surrounding Studies of Susceptible Populations and Individuals. *Environ Health Perspect* (1997):105(4 Suppl):837–841.

16. Snider, D.E., and D.F. Stroup. Defining Research When It Comes to Public Health. *Public Health Rep* (1997):112:29–32.

17. Spicer, C.M. Nature and Role of Codes and Other Ethics Directives. In: Reich, W.T., editor, *Encyclopedia of Bioethics*, vol. 5. New York, NY: Simon and Schuster MacMillan (1995):2605–2612.

18. Goodman, K.W. Codes of Ethics in Occupational and Environmental Health . *J Occup Environ Med* (1996):38:882–883.

19. Beauchamp, T.L. Moral Foundations. In: Coughlin, S.S., and T.L. Beauchamp, editors, *Ethics and Epidemiology*. New York, NY: Oxford University Press (1996):24–52.

20. Ladd, J. The Quest for a Code of Professional Ethics: An Intellectual and Moral Confusion. In: Johnson, D.G., editor, *Ethical Issues in Engineering*. Englewood Cliffs, NJ: Prentice Hall (1991):130–6.

21. Reilly, P. American Society for Human Genetics Statement on Genetics and Privacy: Testimony to the United States Congress. *Am J Hum Genet* (1992):50:640–642.

22. American College of Human Genetics Storage of Genetic Materials Committee. Statement on Storage and Use of Genetic Materials. *Am J Hum Genet* (1995):57:1499–1500.

23. Weed, D.L., and R.M. McKeown. Epidemiology and Virtue Ethics. *Int J Epidemiol* (1998):27:343–348.

24. Coughlin, S.S., C.L. Soskolne, and K.W. Goodman. *Case Studies in Public Health Ethics*. Washington, D.C.: American Public Health Association (1997).

CHAPTER 12

AMERICAN COLLEGE OF EPIDEMIOLOGY ETHICS GUIDELINES FOR EPIDEMIOLOGISTS

Introduction

This document, which is indebted to past efforts to develop ethics guidelines for epidemiologists and to the commentary that has accompanied such efforts, provides the first set of ethics guidelines for the American College of Epidemiology (ACE). These guidelines have been developed primarily for the North American context and thus do not supersede international guidelines nor those developed for a particular region. The background to and rationale for this effort, including the purpose and nature of ethics guidelines in epidemiology, have been discussed elsewhere.

Ethics guidelines are not static documents. They ought to reflect the changing role of epidemiologists in society. In addition, these ethics guidelines do not provide a step-by-step method for reaching decisions about ethical issues that arise in epidemiologic research and practice. Rather, they describe the core values, duties (obligations), and virtues that should serve as the basis for the thoughtful reflection and sound judgment that such decisions call for.

This document is divided into four parts. The first part provides an overview of widely held core values, duties, and virtues in epidemiology and provides concise definitions of these concepts. The second part provides general statements of the obligations that epidemiologists have to various parties. The third part is a more detailed discussion of these guidelines. The fourth part provides a summary, outlines some remaining issues, and draws some conclusions.

Part I—Core Values, Duties, and Virtues in Epidemiology

In this section, we define and discuss core values, scientific and ethical precepts widely held within the profession, as well as duties and virtues in epidemiology. We also relate core values to the mission of epidemiology: the pursuit of knowledge through scientific research and the improvement of public health through the application of that knowledge.

1.1 Definition and Discussion of Core Values

Like other scientists, epidemiologists uphold values of free inquiry and the pursuit of knowledge. The goal of science, after all, is to explain and to predict natural phenomena. Epidemiologists not only pursue knowledge about the distribution and determinants of

"American College of Epidemiology Ethics Guidelines for Epidemiologists" originally appeared in *Annals of Epidemiology (2000):10:487–497. Used with permission of Elsevier Inc.*

health and disease in populations, but also uphold the value of improving the public's health through the application of scientific knowledge.

These core values underlie the mission and purpose of epidemiology. Here we are concerned with core values that are internal to the profession of epidemiology. As such, they are more restricted in scope than general ethical principles such as beneficence (which relates to the balancing of risks and benefits and the promotion of the common welfare). On the other hand, core values in epidemiology are more general (and more basic) than ethical rules and norms within the profession such as the need to obtain the informed consent of research participants. (Here and elsewhere in this document, the term research participants is used instead of human subjects, which is sometimes regarded as paternalistic; nevertheless, the term participants may incorrectly imply that there has been valid consent to participate, which is not always feasible in epidemiologic studies.) Some differences of opinion about core values do exist, and core values may change or evolve over time. Core values and ethical rules about which it is possible to build a consensus are reflected in this document.

1.2 Definition and Discussion of Duties and Obligations

Core values, including the above-described basic scientific and ethical values within epidemiology, can be distinguished from duties (obligations). Ethical duties are more general than ethical rules. Duties are those obligations epidemiologists have to various parties such as research participants, society, sponsors, employers, and professional colleagues. Thus, for example, the duties that epidemiologists have to rigorously protect the confidentiality of private and personally identifiable information are more general than the specific confidentiality safeguards (ethical rules) that epidemiologists ought to use. Most of the remainder of this document (Parts II and III) relates to the ethical duties and professional responsibilities of epidemiologists. Also discussed are specific ethical rules that protect the welfare and rights of research participants and help to ensure that the potential benefits of epidemiologic research and practice are maximized and distributed in an equitable fashion.

1.3 Definition and Discussion of Virtues

Duties, or obligations, can be distinguished from virtues. The latter are motivational factors grounded in professional character (e.g., the need to treat colleagues and other parties with respect and courtesy). Virtues are character traits that dispose us to act in ways that achieve good things, whereas duties and obligations help define how and for whom we should act. An example is the virtue of benevolence. Among other things, it disposes us to provide benefits to socioeconomically disadvantaged persons in society. Other examples include honesty and integrity, which can be cultivated by actions and experience. A distinction should be made between societal virtues and professional virtues. In this document, we are concerned with the latter. Professional virtues are those traits of character that dispose us to act in ways that contribute to achieving the good that is internal to the practice of epidemiology. The time that senior epidemiologists spend mentoring graduate students and junior investigators in the proper design and conduct of epidemiologic studies is an example of virtuous conduct in the profession. Virtues are complementary moral considerations to duties. For example, the appropriate attribution of scientific ideas in publications is consistent both with the virtuous conduct of epidemiology and with an ethical rule or professional obligation. Virtues do not replace ethical rules such as those specified in Parts II and III of this document. Rather, an account of professional ethics in epidemiology is more complete if virtuous traits of character are identified such as humility, fidelity, justice, patience, industry, and veracity.

Part II—Ethics Guidelines

This section provides a concise set of ethics guidelines for epidemiologists. Later in this document, in Part III, we describe and clarify these duties of epidemiologists.

2.1 The Professional Role of Epidemiologists

The profession of epidemiology has as its primary roles the design and conduct of scientific research and the public health application of scientific knowledge. This includes the reporting of results to the scientific community, to research participants, and to society; and the maintenance, enhancement, and promotion of health in communities. Other professional roles in epidemiology include teaching, consulting, and administration.

2.2 Minimizing Risks and Protecting the Welfare of Research Participants

Epidemiologists have ethical and professional obligations to minimize risks and to avoid causing harm to research participants and to society. The risks of nonresearch public health practice activities also should be minimized.

2.3 Providing Benefits

Epidemiologists should ensure that the potential benefits of studies to research participants and to society are maximized by, for example, communicating results in a timely fashion. Steps should also be taken to maximize the potential benefits of public health practice activities.

2.4 Ensuring an Equitable Distribution of Risks and Benefits

Epidemiologists should ensure that the potential benefits and burdens of epidemiologic research and public health practice activities are distributed in an equitable fashion.

2.5 Protecting Confidentiality and Privacy

Epidemiologists should take appropriate measures to protect the privacy of individuals and to keep confidential all information about individual research participants during and after a study. This duty also applies to personal information about individuals in public health practice activities.

2.6 Obtaining the Informed Consent of Participants

Epidemiologists should obtain the prior informed consent of research participants (with exceptions noted below in Section 2.6.3), in part by disclosing those facts and any information that patients or other individuals usually consider important in deciding whether to participate in the research.

2.6.1 Elements of Informed Consent

Information should be provided about the purpose of the study, the sponsors, the investigators, the scientific methods and procedures, any anticipated risks and benefits, any anticipated inconveniences or discomfort, and the individual's right to refuse participation or to withdraw from the research at any time without repercussions.

2.6.2 Avoidance of Manipulation or Coercion

Research participants must voluntarily consent to the research without coercion, manipulation, or undue incentives for participation.

2.6.3 Conditions under which Informed Consent Requirements May Be Waived

Requirements to obtain the informed consent of research participants may be waived in certain circumstances, such as when it is not feasible to obtain the informed consent of research participants, in some studies involving the linkage of large databases routinely collected for other purposes, and in studies involving only minimal risks. Under such circumstances, research participants generally need protection in other ways, such as through confidentiality safeguards and appropriate review by an independent research ethics committee (often referred to as institutional review boards in the United States or as ethics review boards in Canada). Informed consent requirements may also be waived when epidemiologists investigate disease outbreaks, evaluate programs, and conduct routine disease surveillance as part of public health practice activities.

2.7 Submitting Proposed Studies for Ethical Review

Epidemiologists should submit research protocols for review by an independent ethics committee. An exception may be justified when epidemiologists investigate outbreaks of acute communicable diseases, evaluate programs, and conduct routine disease surveillance as part of public health practice activities.

2.8 Maintaining Public Trust

To promote and preserve public trust, epidemiologists should adhere to the highest ethical and scientific standards and follow relevant laws and regulations concerning the conduct of these activities, including the protection of human research participants and confidentiality protections.

2.8.1 Adhering to the Highest Scientific Standards

Adhering to the highest scientific standards includes choosing an appropriate study design for the scientific hypothesis or question to be answered; writing a clear and complete protocol for the study; using proper procedures for the collection, transmission, storage, and analysis of data; making appropriate interpretations from the data analyses; and writing up and disseminating the results of the study in a manner consistent with accepted procedures for scientific publication.

2.8.2 Involving Community Representatives in Research

To the extent possible and whenever appropriate, epidemiologists should also involve community representatives in the planning and conduct of the research such as through community advisory boards.

2.9 Avoiding Conflicts of Interest and Partiality

Epidemiologists should avoid conflicts of interest and be objective. They should maintain honesty and impartiality in the design, conduct, interpretation, and reporting of research.

2.10 Communicating Ethical Requirements to Colleagues, Employers, and Sponsors and Confronting Unacceptable Conduct

Epidemiologists, as professionals, should communicate to their students, peers, employers, and sponsors the ethical requirements of scientific research and its application in professional practice.

2.10.1 Communicating Ethical Requirements

Epidemiologists should provide training and education in ethics to students of the discipline as well as to practicing scientists. They should demonstrate appropriate ethical conduct to colleagues and students by example.

2.10.2 Confronting Unacceptable Conduct

Epidemiologists should confront unacceptable conduct such as scientific misconduct, even though confronting it can be difficult in practice. Steps should be taken to provide protections for persons who confront or allege unacceptable conduct. The rights of the accused to due process should also be respected.

2.11 Obligations to Communities

Epidemiologists should meet their obligations to communities by undertaking public health research and practice activities that address health problems including questions concerning the utilization of health care resources, and by reporting results in an appropriate fashion.

2.11.1 Reporting Results

All research findings and other information important to public health should be communicated in a timely, understandable, and responsible manner so that the widest possible community stands to benefit.

2.11.2 Public Health Advocacy

In confronting public health problems, epidemiologists sometimes act as advocates on behalf of members of affected communities. Advocacy should not impair scientific objectivity.

2.11.3 Respecting Cultural Diversity

Epidemiologists should respect cultural diversity in carrying out research and practice activities and in communicating with community members.

Part III—Discussion and Clarification of Guidelines

In this section, a more detailed discussion of the ethics guidelines appearing in Part II is provided. The professional duties and obligations are clarified along with key epidemiologic virtues.

3.1 The Professional Role of Epidemiologists

Epidemiology is the study of the distribution and determinants of health and disease in human populations. Collectively, individuals who practice epidemiology constitute the professional group of epidemiologists. It has been suggested that epidemiology is a set of methods used in a variety of professions and disciplines (e.g., medicine, health services administration, clinical trials, and environmental health). The proponents of this argument have held that epidemiology is therefore not a distinct profession. It is increasingly accepted, however, that a distinction should be made between the methods of epidemiology and those who are engaged in the application of these methods as a primary activity. It is asserted here that epidemiologists are members of a profession. Hence, this set of ethics guidelines is intended for epidemiologists rather than for "epidemiology" per se. Epidemiologists have organized themselves into various national, international, and subspecialty organizations and in North America have established the ACE to further their professional interests in this region. It is for this professional group of epidemiologists that these guidelines are particularly intended.

The profession of epidemiology has at its foundation the maintenance, enhancement, and promotion of public health by better understanding of the determinants of disease. To this end, epidemiologists can be employed in government positions engaged directly in either research or practice, in university research and teaching roles, in private consulting practice, or elsewhere in the private sector. In addition, epidemiologists have a role as expert witnesses in courts of law and in the discovery process.

Although epidemiologists do not need a license to practice, individual members of this profession should be accountable for the work that they perform. Professional organizations such as the ACE have a role in the maintenance and encouragement of professional standards through continuing education and through the development of policy statements and guidelines. (Although there is some overlap between standards of practice and ethics guidelines, standards of practice deal more directly with accepted norms for the proper scientific design, conduct, and analysis of epidemiologic studies and do not cover all important ethical issues. Standards of practice are further discussed in Section 3.8). Although such statements about standards of practice ought to strive to avoid restricting the development of innovative research or surveillance methods, or otherwise hindering scientific creativity and innovation, they should provide a framework in which scientific quality, rigor, and accountability are enhanced and maintained. Scientific excellence, validity, and creativity can be considered epidemiologic virtues that should be nurtured.

3.2 Minimizing Risks and Protecting the Welfare of Research Participants

In carrying out their research, epidemiologists should abstain from conduct that may injure or jeopardize the welfare of study participants either through intentional or unintentional behaviors or actions (e.g., negligence or unjustified departure from study protocols or standards of practice) or omissions. Epidemiologists need to consider and weigh any known or potential risks that individuals or populations may encounter as a result of their research or practice. Consideration of risks includes attention not only to physical risks as a result of direct contact with participants but also to psychological, economic, legal, or social risks. The risks associated with epidemiologic research and practice may be subtle.

No consideration of the potential harms and risks of epidemiologic research and practice would be complete without a consideration of the measures that epidemiologists ought to use to protect personal privacy and safeguard the confidentiality of information (e.g., income and history of disease) collected as part of studies and practice activities. Although the protection of confidentiality and privacy are discussed in detail in Section 3.5, we provide a brief overview here.

Individuals' privacy and confidentiality of information need to be ensured unless there is an overriding moral concern (e.g., health or safety) justifying the release of such information or if such release is required by law. If privacy or confidentiality must be breached, the epidemiologist should first attempt to inform participants of such required infringements.

To minimize risks, epidemiologists should protect individuals' privacy by storing personally identifying information securely. For example, with the use of a unique study number, the names of research participants can often be removed from medical record abstract forms and questionnaires before the forms are given to data entry personnel and then stored separately. Epidemiologists should restrict access to personal information and store this information in secure environments (e.g., locked file cabinets) including off-site locations for any backup documents. To ensure confidentiality of information (including self-reported and biologic data), epidemiologists should gather, store, and present data in such a manner as to prevent identification of study participants by third parties. No potentially identifying information should be given to third parties without the express permission of the participant unless required by law.

A consideration of the potential harms and risks of epidemiologic research also relates to the need to obtain the informed consent of participants as discussed in detail in Section 3.6. Disclosure of known and potential risks should occur before requesting study participants' participation. Risks should be considered and disclosed with respect to their probability of occurring and their estimated magnitude.

Epidemiologists may not always be able to prevent all risks for study participants. For example, clinical trials may pose greater risks (and benefits) for individuals in the treatment or intervention arm of the trial in comparison to those in the control or placebo arm (or vice versa). Thus, the epidemiologist must ensure that the risks are reasonable in relation to the anticipated benefits before initiating the study.

3.3 Providing Benefits

Epidemiologists have obligations to maximize the potential benefits of research studies to participants and to society. The potential benefits of epidemiologic research are partly societal in nature and include obtaining new information about the etiology, diagnosis, treatment, or preventive aspects of causes of morbidity and mortality, and about the costs, cost-effectiveness, and utilization of health care resources. Although the individuals who participate in epidemiologic studies may derive no direct benefit from the research, opportunities sometimes exist for individuals who consent to participate to receive some personal gain from participation, such as when previously unrecognized treatable disease is detected during health examinations and individuals are then referred for treatment. In addition, many epidemiologists are engaged in clinical trials or practice activities that may provide direct benefits to participants.

Epidemiologists provide societal benefits and advance the profession by carrying out studies and improving research methods. Improvements in practice activities (e.g., enhanced surveillance systems) also provide benefits to society. Epidemiologists should use the means available to them to contribute to scientific findings and techniques so as to provide benefits to society and advance the profession.

The potential benefits of epidemiologic research include providing scientific data that policymakers can use to formulate sound public health policy. The responsibilities of epidemiologists to facilitate the development of health policy include publishing objective research findings in a form that can be used by policymakers. The publication of both positive and negative research findings is important, since it helps to prevent publication bias and allows for additional benefits to be gleaned through meta-analyses.

Epidemiologists should submit their methods and findings to peer review (e.g., review for publication). Peer review plays an important role in improving research protocols and scientific reports. Such measures contribute directly to the potential benefits of epidemiologic studies to the scientific community and to society. Contributions to the peer review process, such as service on a grant review panel or as a reviewer for a scientific journal, are consistent with virtuous conduct in epidemiology.

Research methods that involve greater community participation and collaboration are more likely to provide long-term benefits to research participants and to the community. As part of some population-based studies, it may be feasible to impart some health care advantage to the community following completion of the study, such as epidemiologic research that leads to the establishment of a local disease registry or the training of members of a community in basic methods of population research, or a health care services program. Such indirect benefits of epidemiologic studies may be particularly important to consider in planning and carrying out studies in socioeconomically disadvantaged populations.

3.4 Ensuring an Equitable Distribution of Risks and Benefits

A further obligation is the need to ensure that the potential benefits and burdens of epidemiologic research are distributed in an equitable fashion. Persons and groups ought to be treated equally, although the equal distribution of benefits and burdens may be modified by considerations of special need or merit. For example, vulnerable classes of persons in society and those in special need may merit additional benefits (while bearing fewer burdens). The potential benefits of epidemiology extend to all groups of persons in society including those who are socioeconomically disadvantaged. The identification of disparities in health or the maldistribution of health services across groups defined by race, ethnicity, class, and many other characteristics as diverse as age, gender, sexual orientation, homelessness, and rural residence can serve as a basis for health planning and policymaking and, thereby, contribute to improving the health of those who are less well-off in society. Carrying out studies and practice activities that provide benefits to socioeconomically disadvantaged and underserved persons in society is a part of the virtuous conduct of epidemiology.

3.5 Protecting Confidentiality and Privacy

Privacy is concerned with the right of individuals to be left alone and not be forced to provide information about themselves except when, how, and to those to whom they choose to reveal this information. Confidentiality is concerned with preventing disclosure of information in ways that are inconsistent with the understanding under which the information was obtained. Epidemiologists should respect the right to privacy and aggressively protect confidentiality. Exceptions are justified in both epidemiologic research and in public health practice only if there is an overriding moral concern such as a health emergency or a legal requirement.

An individual's reasonable expectation of privacy regarding access to and use of his or her personal information should be assured. The law sometimes requires invasions of privacy, especially under conditions of a threat to public health and safety. When under a legal obligation to make disclosures that invade privacy, the epidemiologist should carefully weigh an obligation to the law against the moral importance of preserving the privacy of research participants. If an epidemiologist must infringe upon the commitment to maintain privacy, those involved should be informed of the reasons and of their rights under the circumstances. A decision to violate privacy should be made only after consultation with administrative superiors, ethics committee chairs, and/or other persons qualified by nature of expertise and responsibilities.

3.5.1 Maintaining Confidentiality

Except under unusual circumstances (e.g., mandated by a court of law), information obtained about individuals during an epidemiologic study should be kept confidential. Protection of confidentiality is required not only to follow the ethical principle of respecting persons, but also because the disclosure of certain information to third parties may cause harm to an individual, for example, discrimination in employment, housing, and health insurance coverage. Identities and records of research participants should remain confidential whether confidentiality has been explicitly pledged.

Epidemiologists should take appropriate measures to prevent their data from publication or release in a form that would allow individuals to be personally identified. Confidentiality can be violated even without the release of personal identifiers such as names or social security numbers. For example, the release of information about a physician in a small town could identify an individual patient in that community even though no name or social security number was given. Therefore, it should be standard practice to aggregate data in such a manner that individuals cannot be deduced without additional information. For highly sensitive information or where there is danger of retribution for having some characteristic, data from research studies should be presented in such a manner that no identifiable person is placed at such risk. Where group confidentiality cannot be maintained or is violated, the investigators should take steps to avoid contributing to the stigmatization of the group or discrimination against its members.

As detailed in the Council for International Organizations of Medical Sciences international guidelines for ethical review of epidemiological studies, information about research participants is generally divisible into:

> **Unlinked information**, which cannot be linked, associated, or connected (even by deduction) with the person to whom it refers. Since this person is not known to the investigator and cannot be known, confidentiality is not at stake.
> **Linked information**, which may be:
>
> > **Anonymous**—when the information cannot be linked to the person to whom it refers except by a code or other means known only to that person, and the investigator cannot know the identity of the person;
> > **Nonnominal**—when the information can be linked to the person by a code (not including personal identification) known to the person and the investigators; or
> > **Nominal or nominative**—when the information can be linked to the person by means of personal identification, usually the person's name.

Epidemiologists should unlink personal identifiers as soon as they are no longer needed. Identifiable personal information should not be used when a study can be conducted without personal identifiers, unless discarding personal identifiers would preclude personal health benefits for the participants. If personal identifiers must remain linked to study records, a clear and compelling justification should be given to the ethics review committee (institutional review board or ethics review board) along with a description of how confidentiality will be adequately protected.

The obligation to protect confidential information does not preclude obtaining confidential information. Confidential medical and other vital records that identify individuals are essential to epidemiologic research and practice, and identification of persons whose records have been obtained may be needed to prevent those individuals (or others who have contact with them) from developing disease or to identify the disease at an early stage.

Recent advances in computer technology, the development of large data sets, and the ability to link different data sets containing personal identifiers have created great concern about our ability to maintain confidentiality of information about an individual's health. In response, various governmental bodies are considering or have enacted strict laws regarding the confidentiality of health information. Epidemiologists should be alert to and comply with state, provincial, and national (Federal) laws regarding confidentiality and privacy, including those pertaining to data sharing or pooling of data.

Recent developments in genetics also have heightened concern about the confidentiality of, and the inappropriate use of, genetic information, for example, using confidential genetic information to refuse someone employment or deny health insurance. Laws are being proposed to restrict how genetic information can be used. Epidemiologists should remain alert to developments in this area. In addition, epidemiologists who understand genetics can make important contributions to the field by helping to establish procedures that will ensure that genetic information can be protected from inadvertent or intentional inappropriate disclosure.

3.5.2 Maintaining Security

In order to assure confidentiality, epidemiologists should use all appropriate physical safeguards (e.g., locked file cabinets, locked rooms) and security measures (e.g., password access, encryption) to protect records from unauthorized access. Backup files/tapes and archived records should be subjected to the same measures. Staff training and periodic audits should be conducted to reinforce the importance of confidentiality safeguards.

3.5.3 Certificates of Confidentiality

In the United States, researchers can further address confidentiality concerns by requesting certificates of confidentiality from the Department of Health and Human Services agency that funded the research (or, if the research is not Federally funded, from the National Institutes of Health). Subsection 301(d) of the Public Health Service Act, added in 1988, provides authority for the issuance of certificates of confidentiality for health research projects. The certificate relieves the holder (e.g., investigators carrying out genetic testing as part of a research protocol) from the obligation to comply with some categories of compulsory legal demands for disclosure such as court subpoenas for individual research records.

3.6 Obtaining the Informed Consent of Participants

The purpose of informed consent provisions in epidemiologic research is to ensure that research participants fully understand the purpose and nature of the study, the identities of the investigators and sponsors, the possible benefits and risks, the scientific methods and procedures, any anticipated inconveniences or discomfort, the voluntary nature of participation, and the opportunity to withdraw at any time without penalty. Institutions view informed consent as providing legally valid authorization to proceed with the research. The focus is on both the obligation of researchers to disclose information about risks and potential harms and the quality of the consent of the research participants.

Investigators are obligated to disclose information that patients or other individuals usually consider important in deciding whether to participate in research. Potential participants in epidemiologic research should be told the extent to which confidentiality can be protected and the intended and potential uses of data containing personally identifying information. Additional disclosures may be necessary depending on the circumstances. Steps should be taken to ensure that the participants (including minors) understand the information provided; obtaining informed consent is a process, and informed consent statements must be understandable to a lay person. Although research participants sometimes receive compensation for their participation in studies (e.g., reimbursement for transportation costs or lost earnings), they must voluntarily consent to the planned intervention without coercion, manipulation, or undue incentives for participation.

Requirements to obtain the informed consent of research participants may be waived in certain circumstances, such as when it is impractical and there are only minimal risks, although review by a research ethics committee is a necessary safeguard. For example, it is not feasible to obtain the informed consent of individuals in some epidemiologic studies and surveillance programs involving the linkage of large databases routinely compiled and maintained for other purposes. Under such circumstances, confidentiality safeguards and other measures should be used to ensure that no harm can result from the research. Informed consent requirements may be loosened or waived when epidemiologists investigate disease outbreaks or evaluate programs as part of public health practice activities. However, even in outbreak investigations, it is often feasible and desirable to disclose information about the purpose of the investigation.

3.7 Submitting Proposed Studies for Ethical Review

Investigators have a professional responsibility to evaluate the ethics of a study and to ensure its ethical adequacy throughout its term. It is also necessary, however, to ensure that studies involving human research participants be submitted for review by a research ethics committee. The requirement that proposals for epidemiologic studies be submitted to ethical review applies irrespective of the source of the proposals—academic, governmental, health care, commercial, or other. Sponsors should recognize the necessity of ethical review and should facilitate the establishment of ethics review committees. These committees may be created under the aegis of national or local health administrations, national medical research councils, or other nationally representative health care bodies. They help to ensure the conditions that safeguard the rights, safety, and well-being of the study participants.

If an untoward event occurs during the course of a study, such as an adverse drug reaction in a clinical trial or an adverse psychological response during an observational study, the event should be promptly reported to the research ethics committee so that they may help to determine if and how the study should proceed.

Protocols for collecting data for population-based or community studies should be submitted to the local health authorities where the study is to be conducted (e.g., state and local health departments in Canada or the United States and ministry of health in many developing countries).

Issues surrounding the scientific review of research protocols are discussed in Section 3.3 (providing benefits).

3.8 Maintaining Public Trust

Public trust is essential if epidemiologic functions, such as disease surveillance, outbreak investigation and control, and research, are to continue to be supported by the public. Trust is an expression of faith and confidence that epidemiologists will be fair, reliable, ethical, competent, and nonthreatening. To promote and preserve public trust, epidemiologists should adhere to the highest ethical standards and follow relevant laws and regulations concerning the conduct of epidemiologic research and practice activities, including the protection of human research participants, confidentiality protections, and disclosure or avoidance of conflicts of interest.

Maintaining public trust is especially important in planning and carrying out community studies. In identifying public health problems to be studied, and their priority for study, epidemiologists should take into account the perceived importance of the problem to the people living in a community after information about the problem has been provided. However, if epidemiologists perceive that a health problem exists but is being ignored or its existence denied by the community, it may well be appropriate to proceed with a study of a health problem (or an outbreak investigation that must be initiated without delay to address an urgent public health concern) while simultaneously working with the community to gain their confidence and support.

Epidemiologists are frequently drawn to the problems of unempowered communities and may require special sensitivity in dealing with them. To promote public trust, especially in unempowered communities, epidemiologists should consider adopting a "participatory" approach to a research project. Involving community members beyond just recruiting them as research participants might promote trust and provide other benefits.

Care should be taken to ensure that community participation in studies does not adversely affect scientific objectivity. The establishment of a community advisory board may be helpful. In planning and conducting occupational epidemiologic studies, it is desirable to obtain input from workers or their representatives.

The attention that epidemiologists give to standards of practice (as discussed in Section 3.1) also helps to maintain trust. The importance of adhering to the highest scientific standards (e.g., by choosing an appropriate study design; writing a clear and complete protocol; using proper procedures for the collection, transmission, storage, and analysis of data; and properly interpreting and reporting results) is highlighted in standards of practice that have been developed in the field. Reports of epidemiologic findings should include sufficient data (in aggregate form) and sufficient information about the study methods to ensure that interpretations and conclusions made from the findings can be independently corroborated by others. Full information should be reported about the response rate and other potential sources of bias.

Measures for the secure storage and transmittal of confidential information (Sections 2.5 and 3.5), including the development and retention of coding manuals, are also addressed in standards of practice for epidemiologists. Similar issues arise in efforts to provide societal benefits by maximizing the potential benefits of epidemiologic research (Sections 2.3 and 3.3).

Other measures that epidemiologists should take to maintain public trust are discussed in Sections 2.9 and 3.9 (avoiding conflicts of interest), Sections 2.10 and 3.10 (confronting unacceptable conduct), and Sections 2.11.1 and 3.11 (reporting results).

3.9 Avoiding Conflicts of Interest and Partiality

It is incumbent upon epidemiologists (as members of the broader scientific community) to ensure that objectivity prevails at every step of the research process. Partiality can arise through a scientist's own biases and preconceived notions about a problem being investigated. Maintaining honesty and impartiality in the design, conduct, interpretation, and reporting of research findings is essential. Truth-telling and objectivity are professional duties and they can also be thought of as virtues.

Reports of epidemiologic findings should be free of distortions that might be introduced by preconceptions or organized efforts, regardless of whether the research was conducted by private or public funds. Partiality can arise when pressure is brought to bear on the researcher by any parties that have an interest in seeing the research results favor their particular interests. Epidemiologists should not enter into contractual obligations that are contingent upon reaching particular conclusions from a proposed study.

Investigators should disclose any potential material conflicts of interest to their study collaborators, sponsors, research participants, journal editors, and their employer. Full disclosure can be helpful in ensuring transparency for identifying conflicts of interests and preventing them. Epidemiologists should take care to distinguish the perceived conflicts of interests of others from actual conflicting interests.

3.10 Communicating Ethical Requirements to Colleagues, Employers, and Sponsors and Confronting Unacceptable Conduct

Epidemiologists, as professionals, should provide training and education in ethics to students of the discipline. This includes the mentoring of junior investigators outside of classrooms and structured learning environments. The goal should be to communicate the core values and obligations of a professional epidemiologist (i.e., ethics guidelines) and to provide an ethical foundation so that students can deal appropriately with ethical challenges that they will face in their future practice.

Epidemiologists should demonstrate appropriate ethical conduct to colleagues by example. Modeling ethically appropriate conduct while mentoring students and junior colleagues is particularly important. It provides another opportunity to offer training in the ethics and science of the discipline. Examples of virtuous conduct in interacting with colleagues include avoiding personal attacks and appropriately citing the work of others.

Epidemiologists should communicate to their colleagues (including those who are in other disciplines) the ethical requirements of epidemiologic research and its application. Such communication may be by direct negotiation of the particulars of issues such as authorship, consent, and interpretation of the results with regard to public health importance.

Addressing and, if necessary, reporting or confronting unethical or unacceptable conduct such as scientific misconduct are essential actions for safeguarding the integrity and reputation of the profession. Such actions have potentially severe consequences and should be undertaken and carried out with great discretion and appropriate consultation. Scientific misconduct itself can also have potentially severe consequences for public health, for health professions, and for individual researchers. In addressing such issues, epidemiologists should give due consideration to the complexity of many ethical issues and attempt, where possible and appropriate, to educate rather than to confront. Agencies, institutions, and research sponsors should accept responsibility for adjudicating situations of alleged unethical and/or unacceptable conduct fairly, objectively, and in a manner that maintains or restores the integrity of the research process, while preserving the rights of the accused and protecting an accuser acting in good faith from retribution and other adverse treatment.

3.11 Obligations to Communities

Obligations to communities are central to any account of the professional role of epidemiologists. Epidemiologists meet their obligations to communities by undertaking public health research and practice activities that address causes of morbidity and mortality or utilization of health care resources, and by reporting results in a timely fashion so that the widest possible community stands to benefit. These measures help to build and maintain public trust (Section 3.8). Providing community service (e.g., providing scientific expertise to community-based organizations) is an epidemiologic virtue.

The optimal time to disseminate the findings of epidemiologic studies is not always easy to discern. Both premature and unnecessarily delayed release of research findings can be more harmful than beneficial to individuals and to society. Study findings should be interpreted and made available to the public in accordance with the current scientific thinking about the utility and validity of the information. Nevertheless, it may be difficult to strike the right balance between the need to cautiously communicate findings to other scientists with appropriate peer review and validation of findings, and the need to expeditiously communicate results to other interested parties without undue delay. The appropriate peer review, replication and validation of study findings, and other safeguards to assure scientific validity are important, but they require time.

Although epidemiologists cannot always prevent the media or other parties from sensationalizing research results, epidemiologists should strive to ensure that, at a minimum, research findings are interpreted and reported on accurately and appropriately. The goal should be to communicate research findings in ways that allow full use of the information for the public good.

Thus, all information important to public health should be communicated in a timely, understandable, and responsible manner. The significance of the findings should neither be understated nor overstated. Epidemiologists should put the strengths and limitations of their research methods into proper perspective. The results of studies in progress should not be reported to the media or others if such reporting could jeopardize the scientific integrity of the study or mislead the public. There may be occasions when it becomes necessary to terminate a study early and release its findings in order to protect the public's health. Early terminations should occur only after due consultation with scientific peers and the study's oversight committee. Reasons for the early release of results should be clearly articulated.

Epidemiologists have an obligation to communicate with communities directly or through community representatives to explain what they are doing and why, to transmit the results of their studies, to explain their significance, and to suggest appropriate actions, such as the provision of health care. This suggests the need for formal communications training for epidemiologists so that they can better communicate research findings.

In confronting public health problems, epidemiologists sometimes act as advocates on behalf of affected communities. Care must be taken to ensure that such advocacy does not impair scientific impartiality in designing and interpreting new research and implementation efforts pertinent to the public health problem in question. Indeed, epidemiologists who advocate should be open to the possibility of changing their views as new evidence or other relevant information becomes available. An impartial advocate should keep in mind that the core value of improving the public's health through the application of scientific knowledge relies on the ideas that the acquisition of knowledge is dynamic and that knowledge itself can improve.

Epidemiologists should respect cultural diversity in carrying out research and practice activities and in communicating with community members. To do this effectively, epidemiologists should be well informed about the history, circumstances, and perspectives of groups within the community. They should form relationships with formal or informal leaders in the community and consider the relevance of the epidemiologic research agenda to perceived community needs.

Other obligations that epidemiologists have to communities are discussed in Section 3.8 (maintaining public trust).

Part IV—Summary and Conclusions

The goal of these guidelines is to provide a useful account of the ethical and professional obligations of members of the ACE as they engage in professional activities and the application and dissemination of information to colleagues and the public. As such, these guidelines identify and record ethical rules and professional norms in the field and should therefore be viewed as normative. However, these guidelines do not provide an exhaustive account of professional duties and ethical concerns in epidemiology. Additional issues that might be addressed in future guidelines, in policy statements, or in standards of practice, include ethical rules and standards of practice for the long-term retention of data in data archives, data audit, and data sharing; ethical issues in placebo-controlled trials; ethical issues arising in genetic research; consideration of the broader social and environmental consequences of epidemiologic research; and human rights considerations relevant to epidemiology.

Although these ethics guidelines focus both on epidemiologic research and on public health practice activities such as outbreak investigations, surveillance systems, and program evaluations, we acknowledge that there are many professional duties and ethical concerns in public health practice that are not directly addressed by these guidelines. These guidelines also do not provide a comprehensive account of professional duties and ethical concerns in epidemiology subspecialty areas such as molecular epidemiology, genetic epidemiology, pharmacoepidemiology, and psychosocial epidemiology. Ethics guidelines for environmental epidemiologists and practice guidelines for pharmacoepidemiologists have been proposed.

Finally, we note that ethics guidelines do not provide the final word on issues of ethical concern. Rather, specific decisions in particular circumstances require judgments made upon reflection of the core values, obligations, and virtues described in these guidelines. Suggestions for improving future versions of these guidelines can be sent to the ACE Ethics and Standards of Practice Committee in care of the ACE national office.

Acknowledgments

These guidelines were prepared by the Ethics and Standards of Practice (ESOP) Committee on behalf of the ACE. The members of the writing group were (alphabetically) Germaine Buck, Steven S. Coughlin (Chair), Dixie E. Snider Jr., Colin L. Soskolne, and Douglas L. Weed. Rosanne B. McTyre served as a member of the writing group for the initial two years. Other individuals including several current and previous members of the ESOP Committee, ACE Board, and Executive Committee and several other ACE members provided helpful comments on an earlier draft of this document. Initial comments were kindly provided by Gina Etheredge, Kenneth Goodman, and John Last.

APPENDIX

Suggestions for Further Reading

Beauchamp, T.L., R.R. Cook, W.E. Fayerweather, et al. Ethical Guidelines for Epidemiologists. *J Clin Epidemiol* (1991):44(Suppl. I):151S–169S.

Coughlin, S.S., and T.L. Beauchamp, editors. *Ethics and Epidemiology.* New York, NY: Oxford University Press (1996).

Coughlin, S.S., C.L. Soskolne, and K.W. Goodman. *Case Studies in Public Health Ethics.* Washington, D.C.: American Public Health Association (1997).

Council for International Organizations of Medical Sciences. International Guidelines for Ethical Review of Epidemiological Studies. *Law Med Health Care* (1991):19:247–258. (Reprinted in: Coughlin, S.S., editor. *Ethics in Epidemiology and Clinical Research: Annotated Readings.* Newton, MA: Epidemiology Resources Inc. (1995).)

Fayerweather, W.E., J. Higginson, and T.L. Beauchamp, editors. Industrial Epidemiology Forum's Conference on Ethics in Epidemiology. *J Clin Epidemiol* (1991):44(Suppl. I).

International Epidemiological Association. Ethical Guidelines for Epidemiologists (draft). American Public Health Association. *Epidemiol Section Newsletter.* Winter 1990.

Prineas, R.J., K. Goodman, C.L. Soskolne, et al. Findings from the American College of Epidemiology Ethics Survey on the Need for Ethics Guidelines for Epidemiologists. *Ann Epidemiol* (1998):8:482–489.

Soskolne, C.L., and A. Light. Towards Ethics Guidelines for Environmental Epidemiologists. *Sci Total Environ* (1996):184:137–147.

Soskolne, C.L., and R. Bertollini, editors. Ethical and Philosophical Issues in Environmental Epidemiology. *Proceedings for a WHO/ISEE International Workshop*, 16–19 September, 1994, Research Triangle Park, NC, USA. *Sci Total Environ* (1996):184.

Weed, D.L. Science, Ethics Guidelines, and Advocacy in Epidemiology. *Ann Epidemiol* (1994):4:166–171.

Weed, D.L., and S.S. Coughlin. New Ethics Guidelines for Epidemiology: Background and Rationale. *Ann Epidemiol* (1999):9:277–280.

Selected Internet Resources on Ethics in Epidemiology and Public Health

Association of Schools of Public Health. Ethics and Public Health: Model Curriculum, 2003. http://www.asph.org/document.cfm?page=782 (accessed 13 July 2009).

Centers for Disease Control and Prevention Public Health Ethics Resources, http://www.cdc.gov/od/science/phethics/resources.htm (accessed 13 July 2009).

IEA European Epidemiology Group, Good epidemiological practice: proper conduct in epidemiologic practice, 2004 revision. http://www.dundee.ac.uk/iea/GoodPract.htm (accessed 13 July 2009).

National Institutes of Health Bioethics Resources on the Web. http://bioethics.od.nih.gov/ (accessed 13 July 2009).

Nuffield Council on Bioethics, Public Health: Ethical Issues, 2007. http://www.nuffieldbioethics.org/go/ourwork/publichealth/introduction (accessed 13 July 2009).

Public Health Ethics Course, University of North Carolina at Chapel Hill. http://oce.sph.unc.edu/phethics/modules.htm (accessed 13 July 2009).

ABOUT THE AUTHOR

Steven S. Coughlin received his MPH degree from San Diego State University in 1984 and his PhD from the Johns Hopkins University in 1987. Dr. Coughlin lives in the Washington, D.C., metropolitan area where he is a member of the Environmental Epidemiology Service at the Department of Veterans Affairs. He is an adjunct professor of epidemiology at the Rollins School of Public Health at Emory University in Atlanta, GA. He was previously a senior cancer epidemiologist at the Centers for Disease Control and Prevention, and an associate professor of epidemiology and Director of the Program in Public Health Ethics at the Tulane University School of Public Health and Tropical Medicine in New Orleans, LA. Dr. Coughlin is an associate editor of the *American Journal of Epidemiology*, and editor-in-chief of *The Open Health Services and Policy Journal* (www.bentham.org/open/tohspj/index.htm). He is the author or coauthor of more than 190 articles and the author or coeditor of several books including *Ethics and Epidemiology* (Oxford University Press, 1996; 2nd edition 2009), *Case Studies in Public Health Ethics* (American Public Health Association, 1997), *A Message of Love, Hope, and Optimism for People Who Are Worried or Sick: From a Human Subjects Research Participant* (2005), *The Principle of Equal Abundance* (Xlibris, 2007), *The Nature of Principles* (Xlibris, 2008), and the first edition of *Ethics in Epidemiology and Public Health Practice: Collected Works* (Quill Publications, 1997, www.books.google.com). Dr. Coughlin's scientific accomplishments include completing the first two case-control studies and the first cohort mortality study of idiopathic dilated cardiomyopathy. Dr. Coughlin's innovative work in the early 1990s on ethics instruction in epidemiology and public health research helped pave the way for the model curricula on public health ethics developed by the Association of Schools of Public Health. Dr. Coughlin was chair of the writing group that drafted ethics guidelines for the American College of Epidemiology. Since 2004, Dr. Coughlin has been involved with an international humanitarian effort, coordinated by the Yvette Flunder Foundation, City of Refuge Church, in San Francisco, CA, the Allen Temple Baptist Church in Oakland, CA, and the Metropolitan Community Churches worldwide denomination to support children in Southern Africa who have been afflicted by or impacted by the AIDS pandemic. In addition, Dr. Coughlin is founder and president of the Indio Center for Art, Religion, and United Societies, a 501(c)(3)nonprofit organization that was incorporated in California in 2008 to provide life-changing and life-saving services to socioeconomically disadvantaged persons and artists in Mexico, Zimbabwe, the United States, and other countries (www.icarusonline.org).

INDEX